W9-BAX-761

Living Well, Dying Well is a splendid collection of stories that bring the beauty of the human connection—plus teddy bears and martinis—directly into the heart of the reader. Several stories written from perspectives you don't expect, captivate you and linger pleasantly on your mind. The book is like a reality TV show in words. It reveals what we can and sometimes must learn about ourselves when confronting the inevitable—as family, friend, volunteer, nurse, doctor, or patient. Hospice is as much about self discovery and reflection at a key life moment as it is about personal care. This book demonstrates so beautifully how important we all are to each other.
— *Jim Baucshke*
Life Story Network

This collection of life stories gives insight into the process of dying. They illustrate how people at the end of their lives continue to pursue their hopes, aspirations and dreams. They demonstrate how, for some, the end of life may be the most important time in their lives.
— *State Senator Tom George, MD*
Hospice Care of Southwest Michigan, Medical Director
1996-2000

My family needed Hospice three years ago. They helped us and our loved one in more ways than we could have expected. We are deeply grateful that Hospice is there for all of us when needed. Brenda Murphy's wonderful book collects the voices of many people who were touched by Hospice. The book is full of the sadness of parting, but it also shows life's true accomplishments, grateful acceptance, and the possibility of gentle transitions. I hope this helpful books finds its way into the hands of all those who are confronted with life's final moments.
— *Diether Haenicke*
Interim President of Western Michigan University

I felt several of the stories in your book were helpful. None of us, doctors or patients, is very comfortable dealing with end of life issues. Several of the stories show others have dealt with these issues and that while difficult they can be managed. I think as a whole the collection puts the fear of end of life issues at a manageable level and shows that they can be dealt with. I think the book would be a great asset to any hospice or oncology unit. The copy you gave us went to our hospital oncology unit.

— *James L. Poth, M.D.*
Santa Cruz, California

Living Well, Dying Well stories bring to life feelings that accompany significant emotional events or life transitions. Everyone present was touched by playing a part in dying experiences recorded by 12 participants engaged with a dying family member, friend or new acquaintance in the case of hospice volunteers. Healed were the wounds that accompany grief and loss within a framework of loving care.

Here are vivid pictures of how people coped with uncertainty, remorse, regret and guilt, arriving at a kind of acceptance, and sometimes finding peace, love, serenity and forgiveness of self and others.

Living Well, Dying Well is recommended for a broad audience. As Mark Twain once wrote, "Life at its best is a losing proposition. Nobody gets out alive." Positive lessons can be learned that add to survivor quality of life.

— *Jackie Wylie*
Bronson Methodist Hospital School of Nursing

Living Well, Dying Well

Living Well, Dying Well

Stories from
Rose Arbor Hospice

~

Compiled, edited and illustrated by
Brenda Fettig Murphy

Harrington Press
2006

Copyright © 2006 by Hospice Care
of Southwest Michigan

"The Martini Man," reprinted by permission of
Brenda Fettig Murphy ©2001

The stories in *Living Well, Dying Well* are true. The
names and other identifying details have been changed
to respect the privacy of the patients and their families.

No part of this book may be reproduced or transmitted
in any form or by any means, electronic or mechanical,
including photocopying, recording, or by any
information storage and retrieval system without
permission in writing from Hospice Care of Southwest
Michigan, 222 North Kalamazoo Mall, Suite 100,
Kalamazoo, MI 49007.
www.hospiceswmi.org

Murphy, Brenda Fettig
    Living well, dying well: stories from Rose
Arbor Hospice. Compiled, edited and illustrated by
Brenda Fettig Murphy. Introduction by Laura
Latiolais. Kalamazoo, Mich.: Harrington, 2006.
    xxi, 154p.
    1. Hospice care—Fiction   2. Terminal care
facilities—Michigan   3. Rose Arbor Hospice—
Kalamazoo County I. Title II. Latiolais, Laura III.
Hospice Care of Southwest Michigan
RA1000.4 .M5   362.13 M9784

ISBN: 0-9789126-5-9
ISBN: 978-0-9789126-5-9

This book is dedicated to my mother, Anna Fettig,
who died before Rose Arbor was built.

Contents

Preface

Dear Friends,

The idea for this book came to me in 2001 when I felt compelled to write about a personal experience I had as a Hospice volunteer. Once the story was written, I realized that other people might be able to cope better with losing loved ones, if they learned more about what Hospice Care of Southwest Michigan is and does.

Everyone comes to grief at some point in their lives—some at an early age, some only in later years. As Mark Twain once wrote, "Life at its best is a losing proposition. Nobody gets out alive." We are all in this together.

But each person deals with the loss of a loved one differently. There is no single way to experience this grief or cope with such personal loss. It's an individual experience. One person can be stunned by it, another can know its inevitability and steadfastly deny it; yet another can accept the loss, go through all the motions, then fall apart completely two days after the memorial services.

Hospice exists to help people cope with their own death and assists survivors—at every stage, before, during and after—in accepting and growing in life after losing a loved one

This book has twelve stories. Obviously, there could be many more. There were twelve rooms in the original Rose Arbor facility when it was built in 1998. We decided that twelve stories would represent the original facility's rooms.

Volunteers, Western Michigan University students and experienced writers, all of whom gathered their information by interviewing families, friends, volunteers and staff in the greater Kalamazoo area, wrote the stories in this book. While each story is based on an actual person, names have been changed to preserve confidentiality.

Each story has a different tone, message, theme and writing style. It is my hope that every reader will find something of personal value in the stories they choose to read and that the stories might help them cope better with their own losses. Blank pages have been included at the back of this book for readers' notes and personal reflections.

Thank you to Hildy and Howard Kerney, Rita Albertson, Jeff Bell, Nadia Steeby, William Zinkus, Gordon Erickson, Bob Felkel, Joe Wessels, Diether Haenicke, Shirley Bach, Tom George, Carol Dooley, Barbara Smith, Nan Harrison, Karen Jacobs, Jackie Wylie, Martha and Jim Hilboldt, Mary Ellen and Jim Poth, Valerie Flagler, Jim Bauschke; my readers' group who told me hospice volunteers should read this book: Joan Burke, Sheppy Douma, Sunny Hill, Norma Smith, Harriet Stephens.

Thank you to the Arts Council of Greater Kalamazoo and to the Burdick-Thorne Foundation for their grants in support of this project.

Thanks to Laura Latiolais, Development Director of Hospice Care of Southwest Michigan who often gave me the inside "scoop" on hospice and was always there to lend an ear or offer an alternative solution.

Special thanks to my husband, Jeff Murphy, who supported me throughout this project; he read, edited and reread these stories numerous times and gave me excellent "corrective" literary advice.

Brenda Fettig Murphy
Book Editor and Illustrator
Hospice Care of Southwest Michigan
October 2006

Introduction

When I began work at Hospice Care of Southwest Michigan, I knew almost nothing about its mission. Both of my parents were then still alive and my grandparents had died long ago and far away from my everyday life. The weekend after my job interview was spent reading everything I could find about the history and philosophy of hospice care. What struck me then and still sustains my passion ten years later is that hospice care just "makes sense" as an option for those at the end of life.

In the confusion, fear and heartache that surround the realization that someone we love has a limited time to live, the expertise that hospice workers provide can truly improve the quality of life for everyone involved. The modern concept of hospice care grew from listening carefully and responding to the universal needs we each have at the end of life: to be comforted in our physical pain, to be recognized in our full humanity and to be treated with respect and dignity.

The hospice philosophy addresses the needs of the whole individual, as a physical, emotional and spiritual being. It also considers the family's needs as well as the patient's. An interdisciplinary team that includes the patient's primary care physician, hospice medical director, registered nurse, home health aide, social worker, and pastoral counselor, together with the patient and family, develops a plan of care that can be adapted to the patient's changing needs. Trained volunteers are available to provide respite for the caregiver and companionship for the patient. Grief support for family and friends is offered for thirteen months after their loved one's death.

History of Modern Hospice

The word "hospice" comes from the same Latin root as "hospitality". During the Middle Ages when travel in Europe was both difficult and dangerous, monks often provided shelter to weary and needy travelers. Many of these travelers were on pilgrimages to holy sites in search of miraculous cures for ill health. This "hospitality" of the monks thus created the first hospices.

The 19th century saw the birth of the modern hospital system designed to care for the sick and those in need of surgery. Those patients with terminal illnesses generally died at home, in poor houses, or at specially established homes for the dying and destitute. Many of these homes were called hospices.

The 20th century saw an explosion in medical knowledge and therapies. One unintended side effect of this knowledge and the increased specialization that resulted from it was the growing sense among practitioners that death was a medical "failure" to be avoided for as long as possible. The extraordinary measures taken to keep patients alive often raised ethical questions about patient autonomy and quality of life.

In England, Dr. Cicely Saunders was inspired by her experiences of working with the dying to develop a new philosophy of care. Dr. Saunders medical career began when she left Oxford University to become first a nurse, then a medical social worker and finally a physician. She believed in systematic and effective pain management. At the same time, her view of pain moved beyond the physical to encompass the social, emotional, even spiritual aspects of suffering. In 1967, Dr. Saunders established St. Christopher's Hospice in London based on three guiding principles: excellent clinical care, education and research. St. Christopher's, considered the first "modern" hospice, became a resource and inspiration for a new field of health care.

Many of the same concerns about care for the dying were being raised in United States in the 1960s. Even before Dr. Saunders dream of St. Christopher's became a reality, she was invited to speak on her research at Yale University. Florence Wald, Dean of Nursing at Yale was much influenced by Saunders' visit and is credited with founding the hospice movement in the United States and establishing the first hospice in New Haven, Connecticut in 1974. Early hospice programs were not part of the established health care system and were led by nurses or volunteers.

Not-for-profit support and government initiatives funded early programs. In 1982, the United States Congress passed legislation creating the Medicare Hospice Benefit as a cost-saving provision after a government study reported that hospice care was considerably less costly than conventional hospital care for the dying. Over time, many states added hospice care as a benefit of their Medicaid programs. Commercial insurances also often have a hospice benefit as part of their employer or private insurance policies.

Hospice Care of Southwest Michigan

In 1979 a group of thirty community members researched the options for compassionate end of life care in the Kalamazoo area and concluded that they were inadequate. They recommended that a hospice program be established. In 1981 the Kalamazoo Foundation granted funds to launch a three-year pilot program and the Reverend James C. Holt of St. Luke's Episcopal Church offered free office space to the fledgling program.

Five years later, Hospice of Greater Kalamazoo became a certified Medicare hospice and moved to permanent office space given by an anonymous donor. This would be Hospice's home for the next twenty-one years. In 1985 Hospice of Greater Kalamazoo became a United Way agency.

The 1990s saw steady growth in the scope of services under the leadership of CEO Jean Maile. The name change to Hospice Care of Southwest Michigan reflected the geographic area served by the agency. In 1998 the agency opened Rose Arbor Hospice Residence, the first such facility licensed by the state of Michigan to care for those patients who have no caregiver or need palliative care in a more structured setting.

Since 2000, Hospice Care of Southwest Michigan has worked to expand its services to meet the needs of the community. Six additional patient rooms were added to Rose Arbor in 2002. An innovative children's grief program called *Journeys* was added to the extensive grief support offerings. Complementary therapies, including music therapy and massage therapy, have also been introduced.

Rose Arbor Hospice Residence

The results of a study completed in 1994 by Western Michigan University's Service Quality Institute found an *"overwhelming need and support"* in the community for a hospice residential care facility. Ms. Maile knew that terminally ill individuals who did not have family or friends to care for them had limited choices and were not likely to be able to remain at home. A hospice residential facility would provide a comfortable home like environment with 24-hour care. The local architectural firm of Diekema Hamann turned the vision that Ms. Maile and the board of directors developed into twelve airy and spacious rooms designed for patient comfort and privacy. Patient rooms are equipped with sofa beds so family members can stay overnight. Three gathering rooms create quiet and comfortable retreats in which visiting family and friends can talk or share a meal when they are not with their loved one. A special whirlpool bath for patients soothes and relaxes. The small chapel provides a peaceful spot for reflection and prayer. Six additional rooms were added in 2002 making the total number of rooms in the present facility eighteen. Since it opened in July 1998, Rose Arbor has cared for more than 1,400 patients and their families.

Today there are over 4,000 hospice programs serving approximately 1.2 million individuals and families in the United States. Despite these numbers, there are many in our community and throughout the United States who could benefit from hospice care, but are not receiving it. They may be unaware that such services exist or their health care providers may not have talked to them about hospice. Many families who do use hospice comment that they wish that they had started services earlier. Although the Hospice Medicare Benefit defines hospice care as appropriate for the last six months of life, the median length of service is only twenty-two days for hospice patients and over one-third of patients receive care for seven days or less.

In telling the stories of the twelve individuals and their loved ones in this book, we hope to illuminate for readers the difference that hospice care can make for those with a limited time to live. Every day our patients give us the privilege of helping them live in as much comfort, peace and joy as possible until their life journey ends.

~

This book was made possible by the creativity, hard work and dedication of Brenda Fettig Murphy, Kalamazoo volunteer and artist. Brenda was inspired by her experience as a hospice volunteer to initiate the project and then see it through to completion. She brought together a varied and enthusiastic group of writers, volunteers, staff and patient family members to craft a sampling of experiences with Hospice Care of Southwest Michigan. Brenda also obtained grants from the Arts Council of Greater Kalamazoo and the Burdick-Thorne Foundation to make publication possible. In addition to all of these efforts, Brenda created the drawings that evoke the mood of each story.

Hospice Care of Southwest Michigan is deeply grateful for Brenda's generous gift of time, skill and determination to this project. Without her the stories contained in Living Well, Dying Well would never be heard.

Laura Latiolais
Director of Community Relations & Development
Hospice Care of Southwest Michigan
www.hospiceswmi.org
October 2006

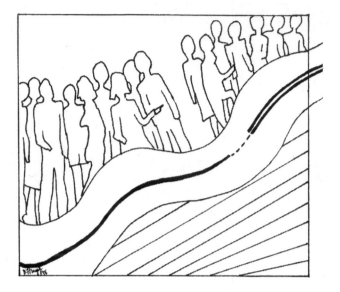

A Friend Departed
by Patrick Crandell

My friend is dead. Staring at his body in that wooden box, I wonder what his coffin is made of. Pine or oak? Does the family pick out the type of wood or does it only come in one type? What an inane question for a funeral. Who thinks about wood when a friend dies? I do. He was my age and now he's dead. A familiar face, another, and another— all strenuously avoiding eye contact, save for one or two who appear to have set aside their preconceived notions of funerals. Death certainly draws a crowd. It looms, daring someone to challenge its audacity to take this life. A pause, a brief silence, all heads turn in unison—Luke's parents. They're good people; they should be smiling, not burying their son. They move forward, nodding and making eye contact with as many as possible. Solemn looks, saddened smiles, heads bowed in reverence greet them as they sit. The priest stands and invokes God. I hope it helps. Something good is gone but I can remember from where he came. The priest fades.

I attended a private Christian school, while Luke attended a public middle school. We met in one of my many vain attempts at socialization. I had decided to join the Cub Scouts because I wanted a friend. Friendship was a difficult concept to fathom when my class had a total of seven members, five of whom found me strange and the seventh of whom appeared stranger than I felt. Luke being my age, my size, and close enough for me to grab a hold of, was immediately affixed the title of "friend". We joined the ranks of Pack 601, and became members of the Panther Den. Luke's dad became our Den leader and my mom became our Den mom. Luke and I sealed our friendship with blue button-up shirts which begged to be arrayed with patches and pins proclaiming our bravery and courage. I wish I could say that we were inseparable, that we were confidants, that we even saw each other more than once a week, but we didn't. I was still an introvert, and he still attended another school. But we were friends.

Cub Scouts taught me much, mainly that I had little common sense, and that I had better get some if I intended to survive until maturity. Scouts promoted teamwork and the value of trusting my teammates, my Den. Our team had many group projects; some we accomplished marvelously, and some when we barely managed to escape death, or even worse, embarrassment in front of our peers. We were men or, at least, on our way to becoming men. The best times were spent relying on each other to pull us out of whatever trouble we had managed to create. We built a bond through numerous accidents and maturity lessons. We were comrades and, regardless of what lay ahead, friends—I assumed—maybe best friends. But feelings change, interests diverge, girls appear, and high school brings experiences never before considered.

I continued attending my middle school and Luke, his. Our friendship varied as our interests did; I continued my scouting days and Luke moved on to new endeavors. When I finally transferred to the public high school, our relationship had changed. I had moved away from my friend, save for a recollection of times spent burning and building, but our bond was not to die so easily. In the few remaining months of my sophomore year, I stumbled into the brilliant idea of running for student council. The kids involved in the council were mostly popular peers with too much money to spend and too many empty spaces on their resume to fill. I wanted to be part of this. Election Day came and I noticed that Luke's name appeared on the ballot next to mine. About that time he walked up and smiled. He asked if I had voted yet, which I had not, and told me he hoped that I would vote for him. Since you could vote for multiple candidates I felt guilt-free about voting for myself, and then for him. He smiled again, and continued on his way. I watched him approach more than ten people during the forty-five minute lunch period. He inquired about their day, wished them well, and reminded them to vote for student council. Perhaps his motives were more selfish in nature. Perhaps he felt he could sway people with his charming demeanor. However, I felt that he believed he could make a difference, and I have always respected him for it. He won. I did not.

High school continued, our lives progressed, little changed. Graduation came. Luke and I hugged, posed for a picture and talked about the future. Future! Ha!

Luke and I graduated from high school, having had only casual conversations as we passed each other in the hall. I assumed that our friendship would always exist, that we could someday go back and speak as if no time had passed. I was mistaken. A few months after I began my freshman year of college, I got a call from my mother. She told me that Luke had been admitted to the hospital, and they thought he had a brain tumor.

The news shook me. Not a simple cold shake, but a blood-chilling, change-my-life-in-a-second shiver. This may appear an exaggeration, but when society says the young believe they are invincible, society is right. My head clouded—I couldn't think. Suddenly life seemed different now that one of my own had been struck down. This wasn't a case of a blotchy piece of skin or even a discolored extremity; this was a burrowing, life-sucking tumor, and it was killing someone I knew. I was afraid. It's amazing how quickly the memories slammed back into me. All those times we worked together or laughed together, only to be contrasted with the instances where I had gone out of my way to avoid meeting him. Regret consumed me. My mom suggested I come home and try to see him, but I couldn't. I let my schoolwork and my social life distract me. Partly I think I was ashamed; mostly I think I was afraid. If I stared into the face of death, I feared it would stare back. My life would be permanently changed, and I was not prepared for it. So I did what most people do in this situation: I avoided the issue. I buried myself in work, studies, and completely mindless and irrelevant activities.

This behavior worked for several months. I almost succeeded in effectively blocking Luke from my thoughts. But there were still times where the thought of Luke lying somewhere in a hospital bed brought back that cold shiver. At those times I tried to convince myself that he would get better and my worrying would only bring me down. So I'd go back to my daily routine. Some friend I was. Then my mother called again, four months after the first phone call. She said they weren't sure how much longer Luke had, and if I wanted to see him, I needed to go now. My fantasy collapsed. I could no longer deny the inevitable: my friend would die, and no amount of wishing could prevent that. I had to see him. A week later I made the trip home. I hoped and prayed that I could handle this and that it wouldn't affect me. But I already knew it had.

The drive to Rose Arbor was about an hour. I felt as though I were traveling to the end of the world. One moment I wanted to be there; the next I wanted to run in the opposite direction as far and fast as I could. I was petrified, but I pulled in to the visitors' parking lot in front of the building. The fall afternoon was bright and crisp, and my friend was inside, dying.

I entered through the front doors and walked down the hall to Luke's room. I secretly hoped and prayed for a fire or a bomb threat or a nuclear holocaust, anything to keep me from traveling down the end section of hallway. Finally I stood before the door to his room. This was it. I couldn't turn back now. I had to continue. There were voices coming from inside. I knocked softly and entered the room.

Then, everything changed.

Luke lay in bed, surrounded by his family, and they were all smiling. Why were they smiling— didn't they understand he was dying? I wanted to scream, cry, run, anything to make them understand. But I didn't. I smiled back.

Luke was bald, and his head a rather different shape. It had a smallish lump on the right side. It took me several moments to realize this was the tumor. He seemed smaller, meeker, no longer the robust person who had a heart to change things, no longer quite the carefree youth I remembered.

"Hey, Luke, I thought I'd come say hello." I stammered.

Luke smiled at me. Then his smile broadened, although it seemed pained from months of chemotherapy and radiation and sleepless nights. He thanked me for coming; he appreciated the chance to get to see me. I felt sick with guilt. I had put off making this trip for months. I had avoided him for so long, and now, he welcomed me with open arms. I felt unworthy. We talked for a while, catching up on what each of us had been doing. I had spent a year trying to discover my future, to learn where my next path lay. He had spent the year living his present. As we spoke my tension and guilt eased away. I no longer stared at the shadow of a man I had known, but appreciated my friend who was still very much alive.

Luke laughed and joked, told me stories of his trials and his joys. He had repaired his relationship with God, something that had plagued him prior to his illness. He never quit smiling. He must have been in such pain, but he didn't let it bother him. Luke seemed very much at peace. He felt optimistic about recovery. He had even registered for college the next semester. I was shocked, but I said nothing.

After half an hour of talk, he directed my attention to a previously unnoticed wall opposite his bed. It was covered with posters, and these posters were covered with names. I was taken aback—almost breathless. Many of my fellow classmates and friends had already been there. They had taken my path and had arrived here despite themselves. They had left encouragement, praise, verses, poems, all dedicated to the young man across from me. Luke's cancer, while seemingly senseless, had affected many very different people.

While Luke lay in that bed, before my arrival, I had questioned the reason for such a good person being afflicted with such a terrible disease. One look at Luke's wall, together with his smile, showed me that while bad things happen to good people, there is always a higher purpose, even if it isn't readily apparent. I now know that life brings sudden changes and we must be ready to face them, no matter how fearful we are. Luke knew this and was ready for whatever lay ahead. I felt like I wanted to cry. We talked for a while longer. I added my name to the posters as another link in the chain of support for this brave young man. I wished him a speedy recovery, and left.

I went home and awaited news. One month later I once again received a phone call from my mother. Luke had died.

The priest closes with a prayer and invites any who wish to follow the motorcade to the cemetery. I glance at the open casket. shake my head and walk towards the door. Did it really mean anything? Was there even a purpose!? WHY! I understand that Luke was at peace and I understand that he brought me to realize life brings sudden changes. I understand his pain has ended, but why. I want to scream. I want to run. I want to rage at the injustice, but I can't. So I leave. As I step outside into the cold winter air, my head clears, and the same thoughts I had after I left the hospice return. My friend is dead, but still he remains.

A Friend Departed

off

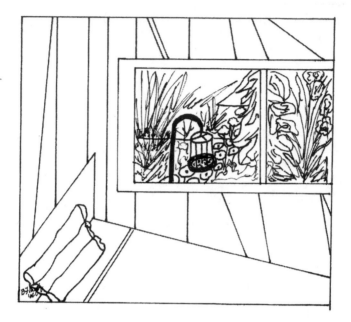

Life in Death
by Elizabeth Cook Seering

Jeanne Dunn sits alone in a booth drinking coffee as the chilly February wind pounds against the windows of the little restaurant. Her salt and pepper hair is cropped short in a pixie cut reminiscent of Audrey Hepburn and she has dressed her small, athletic frame in a cherry-red fleece pullover and black knit leggings. A playful bracelet made of bright blue buttons slips down her arm as she stands to greet me.

"It's so nice to finally meet you," Jeanne tells me in her warm, inviting manner.

"You too," I respond a bit excitedly. The cash register rings noisily behind me, as if it senses my anticipation.

I slide into the booth fumbling with my jacket and it dawns on me that I never told Jeanne what I looked like or would be wearing—she just knew. But somehow looking back on our interview, this comes as no surprise. Jeanne has an unusual ability to connect with people on a more immediate level than most.

The waitress stops at our booth to see if she can bring us anything.

"Just water, please," I tell her.

The water goes untouched for the next hour.

Jeanne and I make small talk about the weather and our mental states, trying to overcome the awkwardness that persists when two people meet for the first time. A silence momentarily ensues and we both smile at each other, not sure who should speak next. Since I am the interviewer, I take the lead and dive right in, saying, "So, tell me how you came to be a nurse at Rose Arbor." The lounge music comes through the speaker above our table as she relaxes into storytelling mode.

Jeanne begins: "I was working in Kenya for three years in charge of a medical ward at a missionary hospital. There was a lot of death there; at least one person would die every day. The nurses I worked with told me I ought to work in hospice care since I was so good with people who were dying. I had never really considered it. But, when I came back to the United States, I decided working in a hospice might be the right fit for me. So, I began working at Rose Arbor in November of 1999 and have loved every minute."

How someone can "love" working in what seems like a very morbid profession, I wonder. "It seems like a very difficult line of work to go into, how do you do it?"

Jeanne answers "Here's how I see it: death and birth are very similar. They are both very personal and can be very beautiful. It's an honor and privilege to be a part of the next step in the natural process of life."

"Well, tell me, how do you like working at Rose Arbor?"

"Oh, I love it. It's such a wonderfully peaceful environment and I have the time to actually establish relationships with our clients, which is what they deserve. Families are encouraged to be a part of the client's life. So many times people come to us from a hospital where their families didn't feel like they could take part. Rose Arbor really gives people a chance to connect with their loved one and be educated on the benefits of hospice care."

There seemed to be more to Jeanne then first met the eye. She certainly had an infectious *joie de vivre*, but I felt there was something to be learned from her.

"So, what have you learned from your work?"

"I've learned to set apart my goals and desires and to think of the other person, allowing them to fail and make mistakes. I feel like a mother in some ways and just want to encourage them, but sometimes their choices are different than I would hope. One thing I have learned from co-workers and other disciplines, like the chaplain or social workers, is to always try to meet the patient's needs. Whatever they want, I just need to be there for them."

Throughout our conversation, Jeanne exuded a warmhearted glow, a testimony to her love of the job. Although my gut feeling was I already knew the answer to this next question, I ask, "Why did you decide to contribute to this book?"

Without having to even think about it, Jeanne replies, "Education. The more people know about hospice care, the less suffering there will be as people live their final days. A lot of people think hospices are just for those who have cancer and some even see it as a death wish, like if you finally allow yourself to be put into a hospice, you are giving in to death. But there is no reason anyone, clients or their families, should suffer."

A solid understanding of Jeanne's motivations for being involved in hospice care had been established. Now it seemed a good time to get to the heart of why we are doing this interview.

"Jeanne, you know we talked on the phone about one particular patient—please tell me about Agnes."

She smiles. "Agnes was a memorable patient. She was very close to my age, around forty-six or so. Anyone could see she was a highly motivated individual and an excellent worker. But she was very angry," Jeanne says as her eyes hover on an invisible spot above my head.

"I remember times that I worked with Agnes on the night shift. She would open the closet and throw things out of it, all over the room. She was this powerful executive who had lived a fast-paced life in Chicago with everything at her fingertips and now here she was in this dinky little town of Kalamazoo. Most of the time, I would just let her throw things around until she was physically exhausted enough to sleep—she just had to work through it."

"It must have been challenging to work with her."

"It was hard," Jeanne agreed. "She was so angry at her mother for putting her in Rose Arbor. She would often yell at her mom. But her mom was just trying to do the best thing she could for her."

"You said she was an executive. Do you know what she did for a living?"

"Exactly, no. But I do know she used to go out and make money for organizations. Agnes grew up in Kalamazoo," Jeanne went on, answering questions before they were even asked. "She was tall. I could tell she must have been very beautiful at one time. The chemotherapy caused her hair to fall out; she was gaunt from all of the weight she lost. Despite her appearance, I could tell that she was a very strong and very opinionated woman. But no matter how much anyone did for her, nothing was good enough and she absolutely hated being at Rose Arbor."

"Why was that?" Rose Arbor seemed to be a wonderful facility. It seemed incomprehensible to me that anyone would hate being there, especially someone who only wanted the best.

"Agnes was used to Chicago and action, and pretty quickly this independent woman had to depend on us for everything, even eating. A lot of people who come to Rose Arbor have to make that transition, and Agnes did it in an angry manner."

"How long was she at Rose Arbor?"

"It couldn't have been more than six weeks, maybe two months. It wasn't a terribly long time.

Agnes was a person that you might say walked on life's edges—a challenger, a go-getter. She wanted the best. Of course, this made it more difficult for her to be at Rose Arbor than most of my other patients."

"If Agnes was such a hard case, why did you want to talk about her? Despite what you have already told me, it seems that she must have impacted you in a positive way."

Jeanne's face spreads into a warm grin. "It was her transformation," she says, as her delicate fingers trace the rim of her coffee cup, her eyes lost in the rich liquid as her mind relives the memory.

"Her transformation?"

"Yes, right before she passed on, a peace came over her. You know, when you see someone so angry, it's hard to be around them. There's no trust because they're struggling so much. But when Agnes made her transition, it was so peaceful. We were all really grateful for that. She was so relaxed."

"What do you think might have accounted for her change?"

Jeanne goes on: "Well, there are a few reasons. When people fight against something for so long, they eventually wear themselves out physically. Agnes, in particular, eventually realized this was not something we were doing to her. It was just the end of her life. Finally understanding this helped her out a great deal, which in turn made her emotionally healthy. Spiritually, she came full-circle. I think Agnes fought because she felt like she had to be mad at somebody, so she got angry at us and at

God. At the end though, she came to peace with Him."

"Do you think Agnes' life affected your own?" It was obvious that it had, but I wanted to know how, perhaps hoping to unearth some formula for finding happiness in times of acute struggle.

Jeanne thought about it for a moment and then answered, "When someone is so strong like Agnes, you have to admire them, and I really admired her. But my heart ached for her. I wanted her to enjoy her loved ones in the last days of her life. When she made such a dramatic change, it gave me hope, hope that every day I can change someone's life. Maybe it's just a little drink of water or a prayer or simply sitting with them, holding their hand and giving them comfort. My time with Agnes proved to me that no matter how bad a situation seems or how angry people can be, do not give up on them."

"OK, so most people would just give up, but you didn't. How did you do that?"

"Anger is something I would rather not be around. It's uncomfortable. I know it's not possible for me to get through it alone. I believe love is the most powerful gift and that comes from the Lord. Every morning I say to Him, 'Lord, I can't do this on my own. Please give me the love and patience I need to make it through this day.' And He always does. This job really increases my faith and gives me the chance to just love people and desire the very best for them."

"So what would you like others to learn from your experience with Agnes?"

"Don't take it personally when someone's angry. They may yell at you, but you need to let them get their anger out. Don't isolate them. A lot of times when we are around anger, we want to get away, but this experience taught me the importance of just being there with them. Every client is a gift to Rose Arbor. They don't believe you when you tell them that, because sometimes it's really hard to receive help from others. I think people need to understand it's okay to let others help them and to feel comfortable receiving help without feeling bad about it," she explains. "My experience at Rose Arbor has been a lot like my time in Kenya. I went there to help those people, but they helped me more. They changed my life. Now I have the privilege of working with people in hospice. When people come here, I am given the gift of establishing relationships with them. Of course, there are times I cry with them, but we also laugh. And in the end, I get the chance to say goodbye, which is so important."

I sit for a moment, thinking through everything Jeanne has just told me.

Jeanne's forehead crinkles in determination as she gives me one last thought, "We are trying to do more education about hospice. Teaching and exposure are very important. When people come to Rose Arbor, they wish they had known about it when their loved ones became ill. The people who come know it's a place where they can be loved and find peace."

I thank Jeanne for her time as we make our way up to the cash register. As we walk out into the brisk night air, I reluctantly say goodbye to this amazing woman I have only known for an hour. She pats my arm, tells me if I need anything to give her a call and then drives away in her little green car. I had gone into the cozy diner expecting to learn something from Agnes' story. I walked out of it understanding the real story was in the woman who told it.

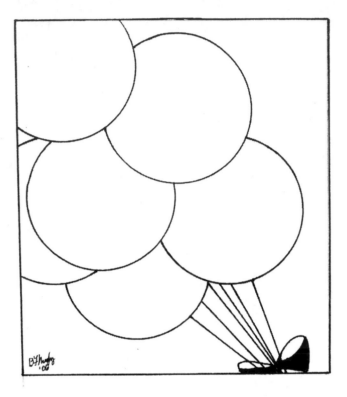

Balloons

by Jan Andersen

I knew Ellen didn't have much time left and that she really needed 24-hour care. But when I knocked on her door that day, I had little hope I could convince her of that.

After having been a nurse for more than 20 years and a hospice volunteer for more than a decade, I'd worked with many different people as they were completing their life journey. But there was something different about Ellen—something that touched me deeply.

When I met Ellen and heard her life story, it seemed so hard and sad. She had been through three marriages, had four children, and at 62 was now divorced and on her own. When she found out she had cancer, she moved in temporarily with her daughter, the one child who still lived in town. But that didn't last long.

Ellen told me, "I figured I'd imposed long enough on Stacey and her family. You know, you always feel beholden and you don't really get any privacy."

Her daughter helped her search for a convenient apartment. They found that, with some federal housing assistance, Ellen could get into an apartment in a high-rise downtown. A beautiful, cozy one-bedroom happened to be available on the top floor, and Ellen headed straight for it and a great view of the city.

Ellen was ecstatic in her new place, and for the first couple of weeks she was fine. She was still able to get around, fix a little something to eat, take naps, read and watch TV. But she quickly found out she really couldn't take care of herself properly living on her own. She didn't have any visiting nurse care, and her family just couldn't do everything she needed.

The way I had heard it, a friend who was visiting her one day suggested hospice. At first Ellen resisted, but she finally agreed. That's when I became Ellen's hospice volunteer.

The first time I went to her apartment, Ellen was still able to get up and answer the door. But within two weeks, when I knocked on the door there would be no answer. I'd gently push the door open and would find her in her pajamas, all wrapped up in a big blanket, sitting in a chair. There was nobody there to fix her meals, so I'd bring her food. She was always grateful, even though she couldn't eat much.

Other than the television, Ellen didn't have many activities. So for some reason—I still don't know why—I started reading *Traveling Mercies* by Anne Lamott out loud to her. That perked her up. She would laugh and get angry all at the same time. Then she'd tell me, "Just one more page, then that's enough for today." And, of course, we'd always go beyond that one more page!

After about three weeks of this, I could see she was really starting to slide downhill. She was trying to do the inner work she needed to do to let herself go, but she was still trying to control and be responsible for her everyday life.

"Can you go on like this?" I finally asked one day.

"Yes. I've always wanted a place all my own," she responded emphatically. "I've never had it. This is mine and I'm going to stay here until they carry me out feet first."

Every time I went to see her after that conversation, I got the same story—that she loved her apartment and how perfect it was. I remember saying to myself, "Methinks the lady doth protest too much."

One day I said to her, "Ellen, this may sound like a dumb question, but you keep telling me that you never want to be anywhere but here. Have you ever even thought about Rose Arbor or someplace else where you could get around-the-clock care?"

She exploded with more energy than I thought she had left in her. "It's so expensive. How can I possibly even think about it? Here at least I'm getting some help with the rent and I know they can't throw me out!"

"But what if that wasn't a problem?" I persisted. "Would you even think about it?"

"I've never thought about it because it's completely out of the question." she said flatly. "There's no point thinking about it."

At last, I thought I understood what was really bothering her.

Looking back, I think she felt lucky to have found the rent-subsidized apartment and didn't believe any other option was available to her. She had to make the best of the situation, even if it didn't allow her to have the care she needed.

But I just couldn't accept that finances were the only thing keeping her from the care she needed. I knew Rose Arbor charged room and board on a sliding scale. And I had seen many people stay there because of private insurance benefits or family members helping out. But these either weren't available or wouldn't be enough in Ellen's case.

I was very frustrated as I left her apartment that day. There *had* to be some way to make it work for her. I stopped at the hospice office on my way home and talked with the director.

After describing Ellen's situation, I asked her, "Can anything be done?"

"Well, we do receive charitable donations," she said with a smile. "Actually, this is exactly the kind of thing we use them for."

The next day, as I was riding up the elevator to Ellen's apartment, I was mentally rehearsing all the arguments I could make to convince her to move to Rose Arbor. I took a deep breath, knocked on her door and walked in. We exchanged our usual pleasantries and I sat down.

Using the best assertive tone I could muster I said, "Remember what we talked about the other day—well, it's okay, you can go to Rose Arbor. Here's how we're going to do it." I outlined the plan that the director and I had discussed the night before.

Well, it was over as soon as I finished explaining how things would work financially. She didn't need any persuading at all. Ellen was so ready to let go of the apartment, it was almost scary. She left everything the way it was and let them wheel her right out of there. She didn't wait for anything, not even her watch or her favorite pajamas.

They took her straight to Rose Arbor right away and as they wheeled her in, I'll never forget the look on her face.

"I'm home," she said, with a glow that lit up the whole lobby.

Of course, she loved it there. I continued to see Ellen at Rose Arbor and we kept working our way through the Lamott book. The next week I took her outside onto the patio a couple of times.

On one of those trips, I asked her, "Is there anything you miss? Anything I can do for you?"

Ellen thought for a moment, then said "There's one thing I would really love. I missed my birthday because I was in the ER. I'd like a birthday party."

It took some work and creativity to pull the party together, but we ended up having a meal delivered in and invited about half a dozen family and friends. By that time Ellen couldn't eat at all. But we helped her into a wheelchair and wheeled her in to her party.

Ellen reigned like a queen at the end of the table. She got little presents and a big bouquet of helium-filled balloons. The balloons were brightly colored red, yellow and blue with glittery metallic designs that sparkled when the light hit them. She laughed and asked questions, and was very alert.

Then suddenly she said, "Someone has to take me back to the room. I just can't stay here any more."

So we did.

Ellen was exhausted, but I could see that she was very happy. She'd gotten the party she wanted. We put all her birthday cards on the bulletin board, laid out her presents and tied the balloons to the end of her bedrail.

When I went back for a quick visit a couple of days later, I could tell she was almost ready to go. And I saw the balloons had started to collapse.

"Would you like me to do something with the balloons?" I asked her. "They look kind of droopy and sad."

Ellen snapped wide alert for a minute. Then she smiled and said, "They're my birthday balloons and they're going with me."

"Alright," I said. "I'll leave them right here. But you're sure you don't want me to blow them up again?"

She closed her eyes and whispered, "No, they're just like I feel."

So we left the balloons where they were. She died a few days later—very peacefully. The totally deflated balloons were still tied to her bedrail.

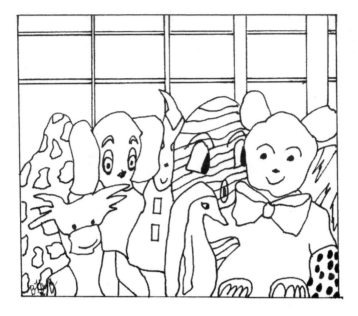

Finding Home

by Dorothy LaRue

Prelude: Anna's Last Day at Home

Life was peaceful as Anna lay on her side watching the fan blades turn, listening to their steady drone and feeling the gentle caress of their breeze. If that moment could last forever, she would be happy to embrace it. The throbbing pain, the weakness and the bone tiredness were but a distant memory as she looked out the window and lost herself in the past. It was just that, though—a moment—and she knew it would soon end. It was time for her to say goodbye to this chapter of her life and to give up the freedom and solitude she had cherished for so long.

Her father loved her dearly, and she him, but he was 80 years old and unable to care for a daughter whose cancer had beaten radiation already. She understood. Her mother had gone many years before and there were no other siblings or a husband or children to look after her.

Her nurse would arrive soon to help get her dinner and medication for the night. There would be the usual, gentle, reminder that the hospice had room for her. She had been hearing those words for months now and, all along, hoping her body would fight this sickness, hoping she would never have to say "yes".

There was no hope left inside her now. She knew it was time to go.

~

Stephanie arrived at Anna's apartment early. She had been noticing Anna's pain increase for the past several weeks and didn't like to think of her suffering alone. Hospice had given Stephanie a key but, as usual, the door was unlocked. That was Anna, trusting and unafraid.

"Anna—it's Stephanie." She spoke softly as she walked up the stairs, not wanting to startle or wake her. Anna sat facing the window, wrapped loosely in a pale pink cotton gown. Her short brown hair and pillow were wet with perspiration.

She smiled at Stephanie. "I must have fallen asleep. It's such a pretty day. How are you?"

"How are *you?*" Stephanie replied. "Your pillow is soaked. Have you been having chills again?"

Anna was pale. She gazed out the window and said nothing. Stephanie had been working with her for five months now and she could tell something was different today. She gave her time.

"Stephanie, I think it is time for me to go to the hospice. Is there still room for me there?"

"You know I've been saving the nicest room at Rose Arbor for you." Stephanie smiled warmly at this courageous woman. She gulped deeply and fought the moistening in her eyes. Anna needed someone strong to help her through this.

"What about my buddies? Can they come?" Anna had a collection of stuffed animals that shared the bed with her and sat on her dresser and chest of drawers.

"Yes, I'll have someone come over tomorrow and pack your buddies and other things. You'll love Rose Arbor. There are big windows, and trees, and birds all over the yard."

She was anxious to get back to the hospice and set everything up for Anna's arrival. "I brought your favorite, chicken noodle soup. Are you hungry?"

Anna nodded happily and reached for the container of soup. The room was quiet as she ate with only the faint noise of the fan blades whirring overhead. A sense of finality hung in the air. Stephanie knew this was the end of Anna's independence but was relieved that Anna was ready to move to Rose Arbor. She watched her eat and took comfort in the fact that tomorrow night Anna would not be alone.

Welcoming Anna

Marie had been a nurse for a long time, and she had been at Rose Arbor for several years. Admissions were always delicate. It was difficult for people to give up what little freedom they had left. Marie was used to approaching the new residents and offering them all the positive energy and affection she had to give.

Most of the time she worked the evening shift. The slower pace of night gave her the opportunity to really get close to some of the residents, and she enjoyed that. On the day of Anna's arrival, though, Marie was filling in for another nurse so she was there at the door to greet Anna.

Here was a small woman with choppy brown hair, tousled but not unkempt. Her large eyes were stretched wide open to take in every inch of her new home. This encouraged Marie because some people were so sad and afraid when they entered that they often looked down or at their caregiver so they could avoid this new reality as long as possible.

Stephanie wheeled her in while Marie held the door and gave her a big welcoming smile.

"Hello Anna. Stephanie has told me lots of nice things about you. Welcome to Rose Arbor."

"This is my girl, Marie, so you'd better take good care of her," Stephanie joked. She often spoke fondly of Anna and Marie knew she cared a great deal about her.

Anna was quiet as she looked around at the warmly lit hallways stretching in both directions and the nurses and volunteers moving about and talking in quiet tones. Straight ahead was a room that had a high ceiling with wooden beams, plush chairs and sofas with lots of cushions, and soft lights perfect for reading. Out the many windows she could see the birds Stephanie had told her about. Ever since she had been diagnosed, she had dreaded the thought of having to spend time in a hospital. She so enjoyed quiet time and privacy; a hospital would give her neither. As she sat there, in the entranceway, with these two women focusing all their attention on her, Anna knew she would like this place.

~

"Would you like to see your room, Anna?" Marie asked. "Stephanie worked on it all morning."

Anna gazed up appreciatively at Stephanie and replied resolutely, "Yes!"

Her room was halfway down the right hallway. She began to feel anxious as they approached the door.

"Here it is." Marie walked in towards the large window and turned to face Anna and Stephanie. She wanted to see Anna's face as she saw her room for the first time.

All of the rooms at Rose Arbor were equally spacious, with two large windows looking out onto the grounds, a comfortable bed, easy chair, sofa bed, and table and chairs by the windows. Stephanie had come in this morning, as soon as the items from Anna's room were dropped off, and spent several hours of her own time getting everything arranged. On the bed was the fuzzy robe Anna's dad had bought her. At the foot of the bed her favorite blanket was folded. Two of the books she was reading were next to the easy chair. And, on a shelf along the wall, all of her stuffed buddies sat, waiting for her.

"Oh, wow!" Anna exclaimed as she saw it all. "This is *really* nice. My buddies!"

Marie and Stephanie smiled at each other as they saw how pleased Anna was with the room. The joy Anna felt was felt by them as well.

Comfort

When Anna arrived at Rose Arbor there was no family that followed close behind. Her father was not always strong enough for the hour-long drive into town. No friends stopped by that first day to spend time with her. When Marie came in for her shift the following evening, the day nurses told her that Anna preferred to be left alone and was very particular about her space.

She found Anna up late watching "I Love Lucy" and asked if she could join her.

"Hi, Anna. How are you feeling tonight?"

"Not bad." Anna was sitting up on her bed with her fuzzy robe on. She continued to watch the TV.

"I love this show. Do you want some company?"

Anna looked surprised by this request and did not respond immediately. Marie could see the gears turning in Anna's head and knew the look on her face. She suspected that Anna was lonely, but also afraid to let anyone get close.

Marie stood in the doorway watching along with Anna, laughing out loud with her big, boisterous laugh. Anna glanced over to watch her laughing. Marie seemed nice, and she and Stephanie were obviously friends. Maybe it would be okay to have someone watch her favorite show with her.

She looked at Marie again and stifled all her inhibitions. "Okay, you can sit down."

"Thanks Anna. I think I'll test out your recliner," Marie said as she plopped down in the soft blue chair. A stuffed tiger with a very large head shared the chair with her. She made sure he was comfortable and Anna watched approvingly. "This is nice. Have you tried it yet?"

"No."

"Well, maybe tomorrow night I can come by a little earlier and help you into it, if you'd like that." She knew that some people don't like to ask for help and got the sense that Anna was one of those people.

Anna replied tentatively, "It looks real comfortable."

Taking that as a 'yes', Marie quickly added, "Okay, it's a plan!" She could tell that Anna didn't want to get her hopes up. Stephanie told her that Anna had been pretty much confined to her bed these last two months.

They watched the rest of "I Love Lucy" together, both enjoying the laughter and the companionship. When it was over, Marie rose from the chair, carefully placing the tiger back on his perch. "Well, time to check on my other residents, Anna. Are you gonna be alright for the night?" Anna just nodded, but Marie could tell she was content. She touched Anna lightly on the arm and, looking right at her, said, "I'll see you tomorrow."

~

Gradually, through these evening visits, Anna began to talk about her life: family, high school days, boyfriends, shopping trips; all of the things she enjoyed doing. She and Marie developed a close bond that was a source of happiness for them both.

Anna wanted her belongings left organized very precisely and Marie was happy to comply. She visited Anna often and always asked what needed to be done in the room. Anna, with her limited possessions, always came up with something. One evening, Marie sat on the floor in Anna's room folding her prized collection of lace handkerchiefs. Her dad had given them to her after her mother passed away. Holding up a pretty pale blue one with lavender lace on the edges, Marie asked, "Was this one of your mother's favorites?"

"Yes, she loved it. I remember her ironing it to keep in her purse if Papa was taking her out."

Anna sat in the recliner, her favorite spot these days. She turned her eyes from the window where she had been watching a fat blue jay intimidate all the other birds at the feeder. She respected the blue jay's ability to get what they needed to survive. Watching those birds every day, she wondered what *she* could do to survive now.

"Did you have many boyfriends in high school, Anna?"

Anna giggled and a slight blush appeared on her normally pale skin. "Not a lot," she said shyly.

Marie pressed on, "Tell me about some of them."

Anna began listing names. "There was Tom. I dated him in senior year. Rob, he was my dad's partner's son. He wasn't real nice to me so I told my dad and he got really mad and had a fight with his partner. They were still friends, though, but Rob never called me again."

She paused, lost for a moment, in her memories. "The one I really loved was George. We met the summer of eighth grade. His family moved down the street from us. They were from Texas, but his dad got a job up here. I used to see him when I was riding my bike. He'd be out riding his bike alone, too. One day he rode over and asked if I wanted to go to the park. I ran in and asked my mom and she said, 'Sure.' She paused, "We had so much fun together."

Marie looked up from her folding, wondering why Anna had stopped her story. Anna faced the window again and held a tissue to her eye. Not sure if the tears came from remembering a childhood love, or wanting her life back, Marie decided not to push it. Sometimes just sitting in silence with Anna was enough.

The physical pain and deterioration were difficult for Anna to bear sometimes and Marie took extra care to tend to her in the ways that she preferred. Marie felt a person nearing the end of a life deserved to have things as they wanted, whenever possible. Anna's wants were not always in line with the way Marie would do things but that wasn't important. What mattered was helping Anna feel good and helping her retain some control over a life unwilling to be ruled.

Unconditional Love

During one of their evening chats, Marie learned of Anna's love for animals. She was arranging Anna's stuffed 'buddies' and wondered how this collection got started. Anna arrived at Rose Arbor with quite a few of these animals, small and large. The family was always growing, too. Nurses and volunteers would sometimes bring Anna a new animal and her dad brought one every time he visited.

"When did you start collecting buddies?"

Anna sat in her chair watching Marie move around, straightening the room. She thought back to her own apartment and what it felt like to clean it.

"When I moved into the apartment, I couldn't take Timmy, my cat." This was the first time Anna had mentioned Timmy. "My dad was too old to take him so he gave him to a friend with kids. The day I moved, he gave me Timmy 2, my oldest and favorite buddy."

This was the tiger with the big head that always sat in the recliner with Anna.

"What did Timmy look like?"

"He was big and soft with orange and white stripes and really long white whiskers. He purred so loudly sometimes it kept me up at night!" Anna giggled. Talking about Timmy seemed to make her light up with energy. Marie was thrilled to see this because as Anna's health worsened, her energy was fading.

The next morning, as Marie drove home, she kept coming back to that conversation with Anna. How wonderful to see this woman, holding on to life as hard as she could, giggling. What could she do to give her that experience again? She thought about how animal shelters sometimes sent volunteers into hospitals with dogs or cats. Visiting someone with a terminal illness was a lot to ask, though. She decided to mention it to several of her closest friends at church.

She explained the gravity of Anna's illness and the certainty of her death. She explained the difficulties of getting close to someone near the end of life. Lastly, she spoke of how the time and energy a dying person shares is truly a gift, quite unlike any other.

One of Marie's best friends, Eleanor, had a big black cat named Marx. Marie had been over to Eleanor's house numerous times and each time Marx ended up in her lap. She was not particularly a cat person, herself. Marx didn't seem to care if people liked cats or not, though. He just wanted love and was happy to seek it from anyone who entered his house. Eleanor was receptive to the idea of bringing Marx to Rose Arbor to visit Anna.

As soon as Anna heard Marie's idea of bringing Marx in, she had a one-track mind. She grilled Marie about him and Eleanor before their first visit and couldn't stop talking about how excited she would be to see them.

Marie asked Eleanor to visit just after dinner; the time of day when Anna seemed to be the most lively. Eleanor and Marx were chatting with Eileen, one of the other nurses on duty. As Marie approached, Eileen came around to the front of the desk and began patting Marx on his head. He rubbed up against her hand, like a dog wanting more attention, loving every second of it. Marie laughed, "Marx won't ever want to leave here, Eleanor!"

Anna was in her recliner. She had asked Marie to set it upright for the visit. She wanted to be as alert as possible. She had been thinking all day about Timmy, and how much she missed petting him.

Now she saw Eleanor, a new face, in the doorway and in front of her, a black cat. This must be Marx, she thought.

"Anna, this is Eleanor. And this is Marx," Marie said as they approached her chair. Eleanor knelt down next to Anna.

"Hi Anna. I am so glad you invited me and Marx to visit with you. He loves attention."

Anna looked right at Eleanor and said, "Marie is my angel. She's here for me almost every day. I told her how much I miss my cat and then she thought of you two." She looked down at Marx. "Is he friendly?" This was her way of saying, "Can I pet him yet?"

"Boy, is he," Eleanor said. "Would you like to hold him?" Anna nodded and Eleanor picked up Marx and carefully placed him on her lap. She and Marie watched as Anna's face beamed and Marx nuzzled for more attention. This was the first of many visits.

The day Marx swaggered into Anna's room, acting like he owned the joint, he won her heart.

She became more alive through her interactions with Eleanor and Marx and began to open up more as well. Slowly, the walls she had built around herself to keep her pain deeply buried began to come down. She learned to trust in the genuine support of those around her and to talk about herself freely without fear of judgment.

~

Marie kept thinking about her friend Adele's two daughters and their sweet dog, Sasha. Sasha was a Bichon Frise with impeccable manners and she knew Anna would adore him. She spoke with Adele about it, thinking the girls could really benefit as well. Sarah and Kelly were fifteen and eleven, and were very mature for their age. Their parents had always talked openly with them about life. Adele saw this as an opportunity for them to learn about the end of life and also to give of themselves. They were both excited and nervous about the idea.

Within a week, Adele called Marie to set up a visit. She dropped off Sasha and the girls after school and Marie was delighted to see them. "O.K. you two, remember Anna is just as nervous as you are. Just let Sasha lead the way."

They found Anna dozing off in her favorite chair. "The Price Is Right" was playing quietly on the television. Marie walked over to her side and gave her shoulder a light squeeze. Anna slowly opened her eyes and looked from Marie to Sasha and then to the girls. She got a big grin on her face and pointed to the dog.

"Can I hold him?" She looked shyly at the girls.

"Sure," they replied, in unison, inching forward. Marie motioned them closer.

"Anna, this is Sarah and Kelly and their dog Sasha." Kelly, the younger of the two, looked intently at Anna, scooped up Sasha and plopped him down in her lap. Sasha shivered a little but sat himself down politely.

Anna immediately started talking to him and petting him. "What a good boy you are. Your fur is so pretty—did you get a brushing today?"

"Our mom said she was going to brush him so he would be nice and fluffy for you," Kelly said, stepping closer and touching Sasha's head. "He likes to be brushed so we do it almost every day."

"Oh! He's very soft." Anna started to scratch Sasha under the chin and make kissing noises to him.

The girls giggled. "He doesn't bark much at all," Kelly continued, "only when we run around with him outside. He gets so excited; he can jump this high!" Whatever fear Kelly had about coming to visit Anna was gone as she gestured up as high as her forehead.

Sarah watched with curiosity, but kept her distance. Marie put her arm around her, "Wanna sit on the bed with me?" The bed was neatly made, with Anna's special blanket at the foot. They sat down by the chair and continued to watch Anna and the dog.

"Sasha knows how to shake hands, wanna see?" As Anna nodded, Kelly offered her hand to Sasha and he put his little paw right in it. She shook it a few times and then let him sit down again. Anna laughed, and clapped her hands together with excitement. "Good puppy," she said, petting Sasha from head to toe. By now, Sarah was smiling too and she gingerly reached out to touch the dog every few minutes, never taking her eyes off Anna.

~

Over the next few months, Sarah, Kelly, and Sasha visited almost every week. Occasionally Adele would join them and she took great pride in watching her daughters show such poise and affection with Anna.

As her condition worsened, Anna received a continuous infusion of medicine. This was an adjustment for her and for her visitors. She sometimes drifted out of consciousness or fell asleep. It was a growth experience for everyone involved. Her visitors learned to look death in the eye, yet still find a reason to smile. Anna learned to let her guard down and treat each moment of her life as a blessing. Though they could not eliminate her pain, the animals were a wonderful distraction.

What Lies Ahead

No matter how at peace one is with oneself and the world, the unknown is a scary thing. Anna was no different in this regard.

Anna had found a comfortable and welcoming place to spend her remaining days. Loving companionship was available to her whenever it was wanted. She forgave herself for any wrongs she had done, any mistakes she had made, and seemed to develop a new sense of spirituality. But she was still afraid to die.

What would she be when her body was no longer able to fight? Facing death had forced her to meditate on what makes a human being, besides just flesh and bone. She found answers in her faith through talking with Marie and a few others, but there were still so many questions. Some of her time alone was spent thinking about possible outcomes for all the unknowns. Meaning was found in past memories and in the new relationships she had formed at Rose Arbor.

She told Marie, in jest, that she was mad at her for bringing so many wonderful people into her life. "Now that I have all these new friends, I *really* don't want to die." Another day, she confided to Marie that her life had been fulfilled as a result of living at Rose Arbor.

In the end, it was the love she felt from Marie, her special visitors, the volunteers and staff who spent time with her that gave Anna peace. As her breathing began to fail and her body began to shut down, she asked for their hands and their hearts. She asked them to be with her—to hug her and hold her and remind her that they were there. During those last few days, Anna was never alone. As her world grew dark, she had a loving friend on either side of her.

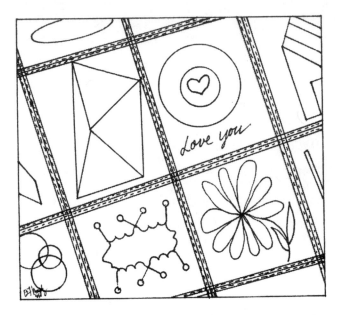

The Quilt
by Elizabeth Clark

For many people suffering from Alzheimer's, it can be hard to recall yesterday while yesterycar's as clear as a bell.

A strange bit of serendipity and synchronicity led to Rose Arbor mirroring the past for one cherished client, which helped make the serene hospice setting an ever more peaceful place from which to pass on.

Rosella would've hated that last sentence.

Even in her later days when Alzheimer's was taking its toll and her memory wasn't up to snuff, she was a stickler for correct grammar and would've shaken her head at a sentence ending in a preposition!

I hope she'll forgive me and note all that lovely alliteration.

Her daughter, Mary, and I met at Water Street Café. She offered me some insights into her mother's life story over mochas and pastries. It was very easy to become enraptured with Rosella.

Mary beams with pride when she recalls her mother's going back to college when she herself enrolled. The term "continuing education" didn't exist then and a 45-year-old woman taking a college course drew curious stares.

You get the impression Mary's bumper might've boasted "Proud daughter of a back-to-school parent" if such a sticker existed.

Not only did Rosella set a precedent for continuing education for women, this amazing lady left a bread crumb trail for other women as she launched the Chrysalis program at Saginaw Valley State University. This program helped many disenfranchised women and non-traditional students to negotiate the college campus and incorporate the university into their busy lives. The Chrysalis program ended when Rosella retired.

"My mother was bigger than life to me," Mary said as she rattled off her mother's formidable resume—teaching English, writing poetry, founding the Michigan Women's Studies Association, assisting in the founding of the Women's Historical Museum in Lansing, compiling an extensive exhibition on women in the circus. Mary recalls her mother being way ahead of her time.

"It was hard to watch her lose her mind because that was her most valuable asset," Mary said. "She had a brilliant mind. We didn't dare say the word Alzheimer's around her. She'd say she was 'getting forgetful.'"

"Eventually Rosella's physical condition deteriorated to the point where she was hospitalized. She couldn't understand why she was there, and felt trapped and frightened." With Rosella's memories becoming fuzzy, Mary couldn't leave her bedside at the hospital because when she was gone, her mother became so agitated that she'd tug her tubes out, get out of bed and try to leave. So Mary slept on the cold linoleum floor in her room and became her mother's constant companion. It was ironic that Rosella, who'd devoted her career to restoring dignity to the lives of other women, could not enjoy the dignity and privacy she held so dear as her life came to its end.

Enter Rose Arbor, a hospice care facility that's as much a godsend to those grieving by bedsides of loved ones as it is a comfort to the clients themselves.

Before securing a room for Rosella at Rose Arbor, Mary had even considered buying a condo so she could be with her mother all the time and care for her. Rose Arbor seemed to fit all of Rosella and Mary's needs perfectly.

While the spacious private room, the view of the woods and the birds flitting about outside her window would provide much comfort to Rosella, it was the hand-made quilt on her bed at Rose Arbor that made her feel most at home.

The Log Cabin Quilters, an association of quilt-makers in Southwest Michigan that donates its crafts to non-profit organizations like Hospice, stitch one-of-a-kind quilts for the Rose Arbor rooms.

Rosella's quilt provided her with much more than warmth.

"You found my quilt," she gasped as she was wheeled into her room. Mary exhaled a sigh of relief.

Rosella had been distraught for some time about her grandmother's missing quilt. She was convinced she'd given it to Mary, who knew for certain that she didn't have it.

Rosella had her heart set on passing this heirloom down to her daughter. Mary was at her wits' end wondering what had happened to this beloved blanket and frustrated at her mother's insistence that she herself had mislaid it. The Rose Arbor quilt came like divine intervention.

"My mother was losing her sight and was blind in one eye," Mary said. "She couldn't see as well as she used to. This quilt just happened to be the colors she could see. Perhaps if it had been the real thing she might not have recognized it."

Rosella was an accomplished poet and a philanthropist who'd think nothing of paying for a stranger's college education, but she did not number sewing among her many skills. She admired quilting and sewing as the highest form of decorative art, and was tickled pink when her grandson sewed her some pillows, which she treasured just like the missing quilt. Her daughter wonders whether any other quilt in any other room would've sparked Rosella's imagination in quite the same way.

The attentive staff at Rose Arbor made certain Rosella was always brought that same quilt, still warm from the dryer whenever it needed to be washed. As its creator picked through fabric scraps of hummingbirds and swans, autumn leaves and wildflowers, choosing each square with love and compassion, could an angel have been sitting on her shoulder pointing to the proper patches?

The quilt wasn't the only attribute of Rose Arbor that wrapped Rosella's last days in warmth. The Rose Arbor greeter's name was Dorothy, and coincidentally the name of an old neighbor of Mary's whom Rosella had befriended. Rosella was sure, however, that this Dorothy at Rose Arbor was her old and dear friend. So, Rosella had her old friend, her treasured heirloom, her privacy and her daughter's hand to hold. All was right with the world again.

The day before Rosella died, an aide helped Mary take her mother to the super-sized tub at Rose Arbor to enjoy a bath. Rosella loved sinking into the suds—her answer to many of life's troubles had always been to "take a bath." Whenever Mary had consulted her mother about any sickness or stress she was encountering, Rosella's advice had invariably been to "take a bath, dear." Rosella finally broke free of the cocoon of this earthly life the next morning which happened to be Good Friday.

Mary still tears up unexpectedly from time to time as she remembers her mother. Luckily, the napkins on the table at Water Street double as Kleenex in a pinch.

And while the Log Cabin quilt that brought so much comfort to Rosella now brings comfort to another client at Rose Arbor, Mary finally has a quilt of her very own. Just days after her mother's passing, Mary was cleaning out the family home and came upon a large box high up in the corner of a closet in the attic. There carefully wrapped in yellowed tissue paper to be handed down to her daughter and best friend was the missing quilt.

It was as though Rosella's hands had reached down from heaven and put it there for her to find.

The Quilt

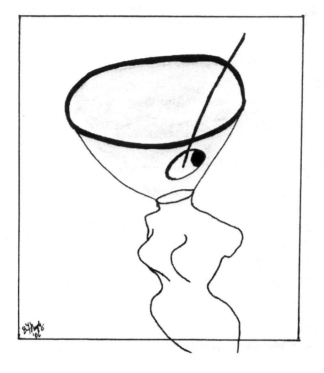

The Martini Man
by Brenda Fettig Murphy

Naomi was the volunteer coordinator for Hospice. She called me the first Friday in June to take on a patient—my first one. Up to this point, in spite of having gone through a rigorous twenty-hour volunteers' training course, I had done only clerical work in the main office or helped serve meals at Rose Arbor, the local hospice facility.

"His name is Sam Wood. I was wondering if you'd like to be his volunteer. He doesn't have too many visitors—he's out at Rose Arbor. How about it?"

"OK, I'll give it a shot."

"I'll send you his file in the mail."

Sam's file arrived the next day. He was 82, a widower with four children, two of whom lived here in Kalamazoo. "Short visits preferred – tires easily." His diagnosis read "COPD" – which meant nothing to me. I looked it up in my trusty *Taber's Medical Dictionary*: "Chronic obstructive pulmonary disease." Basically, it means the lungs function less and less, then finally close down completely and you die.

How do you cope with that, knowing you were going to breathe less and less, and then one day stop breathing altogether? I wonder if he knows what "COPD" is.

I decided to drive out to Rose Arbor on Monday to meet Sam and see what he was all about.

~

I entered Rose Arbor's front door and walked towards the nurse's break room where the volunteers usually left their coats and bags and glanced at the rooms' chart. Sarah, one of the nurses, was sitting at the table in the break room sipping a cup of coffee and updating her charts.

"Hi, Sarah. I see you're busy. I have a quick question. Where is Sam Wood's room?"

"He's in number three. Are you going to see him?"

"Yes, I'm going to be his volunteer."

"That's great—he'll be delighted. Try to do most of the talking though; he gets really tired. He's a nice old guy. . .oh, and he's a little hard of hearing so you'll have to speak up."

Well, maybe this won't be so bad after all. But there was still a slight twinge in the pit of my stomach as I went down the hall to find Sam. The door of Room 3 was slightly ajar so I knocked firmly.

"Come in," a deep voice answered.

Sam Wood was propped up in bed wearing a pale blue, checkered hospital gown. His feet stuck out from under the sheet at the foot of the bed. A face with strong features, a few well defined wrinkles and dark blue eyes greeted me. His hair was very short, curly and white. The chin was stubbly, unshaven yet that day. Rimless glasses perched on his nose. A Pulmo Aid machine stood on his nightstand. Its colorless air hose ran beside the bed ending in a double pronged plug which fit into Sam's nose. He reminds me of my dad, I thought.

The room itself was completely bare. Nothing of a personal nature was visible in it at all. How odd, I thought as I approached the bed. Where were his things? Hadn't he brought anything with him?

"Hi, Sam. My name is Anne Bernham. I'm your volunteer."

"Well, nice to meet you." The blue eyes looked me over from head to toe. "What does that mean— that you're my volunteer?"

"It means that I'm going to visit you a few times a week and keep you company."

"That's OK with me, sit right down. Always like having a pretty gal coming to visit me. Nothing wrong with that."

Hmmm, a take-charge kind of guy. Sam could be interesting. I pulled a chair up next to the bed and sat down. Sam and I talked for over half an hour. Actually, Sam did most of the talking.

He talked about his life. Sam had been in the Navy in the Pacific, and upon his return had married Ellie, his high school sweetheart. They lived in Kalamazoo, but he had worked in Three Rivers as a typesetter for a printing company.

"I did lots of Tony the Tiger stuff for Kellogg. The printing business was real different back then. We did it all by hand."

He and Ellie had had four boys. Yes, they came to visit him and brought his grandchildren once in a while too.

"Nick, the one who lives in Detroit, he only comes once in a while. He's not married, but he's real busy with his work." The words began to come more slowly. All of a sudden Sam seemed tired. His breathing became more labored and he looked a bit wan. I took this as my cue to end our visit before he got really worn out.

"Sam, I'm going to let you take a rest now before your dinner. But I'll be back on Wednesday to see you." I took his hand and pressed it gently as I said good-bye.

"OK," Sam wheezed, "you be sure and come back, you hear?" I went out into the hallway and made my way to the nurses' station. Sarah was getting medications together for the 4:30 distribution.

"Sarah, what's the story on Sam? His room is so bare. There's not one thing in his room that's personal, but he says he has family here and they come to visit him. What happened to all his stuff?"

"Well, it's a bit complicated. Sam was in Bridgeman Hospital for two months before he came here. He was diagnosed as terminal so he was dying. But then, he didn't die. His family cleaned out his apartment and they got rid of all his stuff because they thought this was it. But Sam just wouldn't go. Finally, he had to leave the hospital. He came here five days ago. He actually seems to have perked up a bit since he got here. How was your visit?"

"It went very well. Actually, he talked and talked. I did most of the listening. That's not how it was supposed to be. But he just wanted to talk and I let him. Then all of a sudden, he seemed to get tired so I left. I'm coming back on Wednesday."

"Well, that's not uncommon with COPD. It comes and goes in spurts. You'll have to just play it by ear whenever you see him."

~

On Wednesday at four o'clock I once again knocked on the door of Room 3.

"Hey, Sam, it's Anne. I'm here to keep you company again."

"Been waitin' for you," Sam replied as he attempted to raise himself to a sitting position in the bed. "So, whatcha been doing since Monday?" His Pulmo Aid pumped away giving him oxygen.

"Nothing really exciting. I went out once to practice golf. I'm just a beginner so I need lots of practice. Lots of swings on each hole for me!"

"Well, you just keep at it. You'll get the hang of it. I used to play a lot. Taught my kids to play too. When Ellie and I lived in California, she didn't play much golf, but I'd play almost everyday. Then at 5 o'clock, I'd come home and we'd have our martinis out on our little screened-in porch. Boy, that was the way to finish the day. I sure miss my martini. Made it with Bombay Sapphire. That's a great gin."

"Martinis, eh? They don't serve them to you here?" I kidded him.

"Nope, and I'd sure love to have one."

I suddenly thought, why not? So I asked him: "Would you like me to bring you a martini, Sam? Of course, I'd have to check with the nurse…"

"Boy, would that taste good. Hmmmm, I'd really like that. It's got to be made with just gin and water—no vermouth in it and only a bit of water. That's how I like it. You'd really bring me a martini? You sure are one nice gal, Annie."

"OK, Sam, I'll see what I can do about it."

That afternoon when I left Sam, I went in search of his nurse.

"Sarah, how would it be if I brought Sam a martini? He told me he'd love to have one. Can he have one or would it interfere with his meds?"

"Wow, what an idea." laughed Sarah. "Yeah, I bet he'd love a martini, that old fox. No, I don't think it would do him any harm. Sure, go for it."

~

When I got home, I searched high and low for the right glass in which to serve Sam his martini. After a thorough search of closets and cabinets, I finally found the perfect glass. A friend from California had brought two glasses from the Palm Desert Art Museum shop as a house gift when she'd visited us last year. The stem of each glass was carved in the shape of a torso. One was a female, the other was a male. The female glass' stem was quite shapely and most generously endowed. I selected this one for Sam, thinking he'd probably enjoy drinking his martini from this special glass.

Friday afternoon I arrived back at Rose Arbor, my little red cooler filled to the brim with a pint bottle of Bombay Sapphire gin, water bottle, shot glass, jar of pimento olives, ice cubes, a stirrer and the glass which was carefully wrapped in a linen dish towel. Sam was anxiously awaiting my arrival. I entered his room and put the cooler down on the floor at the foot of the bed.

"Hey, Annie, you've got something in there for me, don't you?"

"Yes, I do, Sam. How'd you guess?"

"Well, that's great. I've been looking forward to this. Now close the door, Annie." said Sam as he started to pull himself up to a sitting position in the bed. "Now you help me sit up," he commanded. He was used to giving orders. "I really want to enjoy this." With that, he attempted to swing his legs over the side of the bed. But his gown was stuck and bunched up around his waist, leaving him somewhat exposed. Sam was completely oblivious to this; he was focused only on the martini makings.

"Let me help you, Sam. Things seem to be a bit tangled up." I said making direct eye contact with him, not looking at his exposed anatomy. I pulled the gown down around his knees, lifted both his legs over the side of the bed and helped him into a sitting position.

"Now, bring that tray table over here so I can lean on it and tell you exactly how to mix my martini," instructed Sam.

I began to take the martini makings out of the cooler. As I unwrapped the glass, it caught Sam's eye.

"What kind of a glass is that? Give it here to me, let me see it." He stared at the torso very closely, slowly fingering its shape. He held it quietly for a long moment.

"That's a very interesting glass—it should make a great martini!" Smiling, he handed it back to me.

"OK, now you tell me how to make this martini, Sam."

Sam adjusted his air-hose nose piece deliberately and settled himself further by propping his elbows on the bed-tray table. His bare feet dangled almost to the floor.

"First of all, put a few ice cubes in the glass. That's it—good—a couple more. There. Now measure out a shot of gin. Fill it up good."

I opened the bottle—a pretty bright blue color, that Bombay Sapphire—measured a shot, then carefully poured it over the ice cubes,

"OK, now pour another one."

"Another shot of gin?"

"Yes, another shot of gin. Go ahead, just do it." I did it.

"OK, now put two olives in it." I put two huge green olives into the glass.

"Now, pour a half shot of water in it." I poured the water into it.

"Now, put a few more ice cubes in it and stir it around twice."

Definitely not a James Bond martini man, I thought. The martini glass was filled to the brim. Sam took a deep breath, carefully picked up the almost overflowing glass, brought it slowly to his lips without spilling a drop and drank the nectar of his gods!

"Ah, now that's it. A perfect martini." said Sam. "You're a great gal, Annie. I really appreciate this." He proceeded to drink the entire martini.

"That was perfect. I can't tell you how much I enjoyed that!" said Sam. "Now, make me another one."

"What?" I exclaimed.

"You heard me—make me another one."

And so I did. We talked and the time passed. When he'd finished the second one, he grinned at me. Sam was really enjoying himself, but I saw his breathing was becoming more difficult.

"How about if I help you take a break now and get a little rest?"

He agreed saying, "Yeah, you're right, I feel a little tired now. This was the best afternoon I've had in a long, long time."

I helped him back into a reclining position in his bed. He closed his eyes and smiled contentedly like an old Cheshire cat who just swallowed a big fat canary.

A knock sounded at the door and Sarah appeared carrying a plastic mask.

"It's time for your inhalation treatment, Sam. Hey - what's going on in here? Looks like you guys were having a private party!" She surveyed the glass, the cooler and its contents.

"Well, Annie brought something special for me. Something I really enjoyed, not like that terrible medicine stuff you're always bringing me," Sam wheezed.

"Could that have been a martini?" laughed Sarah "That glass is definitely something extra special, isn't it? Sam."

"This martini was the perfect medicine," said Sam very seriously as Sarah helped him slide the inhalation mask over his face.

~

Over the next seven weeks I brought Sam his martinis at least once a week. I usually tried to enter Rose Arbor quickly and quietly so that no one would notice my little red cooler. But word spread among the other staff members and nurses. They lost no time in kidding me about my unusual medical treatment for Sam. Meanwhile, his condition remained relatively unchanged.

For each "martini" visit, we had a ritual. He gave me directions. I followed them exactly. Sam loved it. He was in charge again!

One afternoon as he was drinking his martini, he turned to me very seriously and said, "Boy, is this good. You know what I'd like now, to go with it? A cigarette. It'd be absolutely perfect. Can you get me one, Annie?"

"Sam, you've got to be kidding, "I laughed. "I don't think I can do that. You're right. It'd taste terrific, but I think they'd put us both out of here in a New York second."

My God, I thought, that's all he needs—a cigarette. Unquestionably it would taste great with a martini. Somehow those two tastes just go together, but that's probably how he got here in the first place, too many martinis and cigarettes. On the other hand, he's dying—so why not? It certainly wouldn't do any harm, would it? Of course, the oxygen tank in the room might present a real problem. I visualized an explosive exit scenario!

Rose Arbor allowed no smoking on the premises. However, I'd seen other patients in wheelchairs with breathing tanks attached being wheeled out the back door to a cul-de-sac behind the facility to enjoy their "smoke." But Sam knew he was in no condition to attempt a trip outdoors. So he talked about how it was, having that first cigarette, how great it tasted with a martini as the tobacco tingled your tongue and the smell of the smoke permeated the room—but in our hearts, we both knew it was thing of the past for him, never to be enjoyed again.

One Friday I brought Sam a bouquet of yellow sunflowers. They looked wonderful in a huge vase set on top of the TV. He said he liked them. But two days later when I visited him, the flowers were gone. Another time I brought him a golf magazine. We looked through it together that day. But the magazine was gone the next time too.

It bothered me at first, the austerity of the room, the absence of decorations or personal possessions of any kind. I wondered, was it his choice that they were removed or did someone just take them out? But over time, I became more comfortable in the room. It seemed uncomplicated, simple, serene...is it easier to go that way at the end?

Another day I massaged Sam's feet. They were beautifully shaped with long slender toes, no bunions or calluses.

"Sam, you've got nice feet. Do you know that?"

"Yup, I do know that. They're not bad for having been walked on for 82 years, are they? It feels so good when you rub my feet like that—you just don't know how good it feels."

Other days the martini and the torso glass were the focus of our visits. We'd always talk, and he still did most of the talking. Sometimes I'd rub his arms and hands with lotion because they were so dry. As the weeks passed, his arms became more mottled with black and blue marks and blotches, and his breathing became more difficult. But he still insisted on pulling himself up to a sitting position to drink those martinis.

One afternoon when I entered the room, a young man was sitting and talking to him. The young man had Sam's dark blue eyes and short curly brown hair. He stood up as I came in and introduced himself.

"I'm Greg Wood, Sam's youngest son. I live here in Kalamazoo. You must be Annie, the martini lady. I've heard quite a lot about you."

"Glad to meet you, Greg. Your dad's told me about you and your family. And yes, I have been visiting him during the cocktail hour and bringing him his martini."

Sam smiled at Greg and me, leaning back against his pillows. The three of us talked about how life in Kalamazoo had changed over the past 25 years. Sam's spirits seemed very up. I left feeling good too.

~

My next martini visit was three days later, a hot sweltering late August afternoon. It was evident Sam's condition had changed. His breathing was louder and slower. He was sweating profusely. I set the cooler down on the floor, went over to the bed and took his hand. It was cool, but his pillow was soaking wet as were his gown and sheets.

"Hey, Sam, how's it going today?"

"Not so good, Annie. Did you bring my martini?"

"Yes, it's here, but maybe we should get you a dry gown and sheets."

"No, I don't want that. Just make my martini," Sam grumbled, attempting to lift himself up. It proved too much effort. He fell back on the pillow.

I took the torso glass out of the cooler, stood it on the bed tray table and began making the martini. A chair was wedged right next to the tray table. The space seemed oddly cramped and warm.

"You know, Sam, maybe your sheets and gown should be changed. They're really damp. You'd be much more comfortable if they were dry. Hey, here's someone to help do it." A nurse's aide had come into the room to bring clean bathroom towels.

"Can you help me change Sam's gown? He's soaking wet."

"Sure, I can help you." said the nurse's aide. Her nametag read "Janet."

"I don't want to be changed," growled Sam. "I want to stay just the way I am. Just make me my martini."

But Janet and I changed Sam over his protests. His breathing became more difficult. After we got him into a dry gown and changed the bed sheets, I stood next to the tray table, pouring the gin into the torso glass.

Janet came around behind me to replace Sam's water bottle. She moved the chair and reached for the bottle. The top of the chair back hit the tray table hard as she pulled it out.

The sudden jolt sent the martini glass flying. It shattered on the floor. Shards of glass were everywhere. The smell of gin permeated the room. Sam twisted and turned in the bed, gasping for breath, trying to see what was going on.

Oh God, what have I done? Janet stood stock-still, looking at the pieces of glass.

"Go get some paper towels so we can clean this up," I said.

She hurried into the bathroom, returning with two handfuls of towels. We picked up the pieces. She grabbed the waste basket filled with remnants of martini and broken glass, and made a hasty retreat out the door.

Sam turned towards me, beckoning me over to the bed. I'd never seen him like this before. He was very angry. His breathing was quite difficult.

"Now you listen to me, young lady. Don't you ever do that again. You hear me? You do what I say. I just wanted my martini. I did not want to have my gown and sheets and everything all changed and upset. Now I don't want any martini – not today. And don't you ever tell anyone what just happened in here. Now just go away." He slumped back on his pillow, completely exhausted, his face drained of color.

"Oh Sam, I'm so sorry." I began apologetically. "I'm sorry I didn't listen to you. Please forgive me. . . ."

Sam closed his eyes and turned away.

I hurried from the room, my eyes filling with tears. I ran to the nurses' break room which luckily was empty. And I cried. I felt absolutely awful. My job here was to make people feel better, not get them angry and upset. How could I have been so insensitive? I didn't listen to him when he told me what he wanted. His condition had changed drastically, but I hadn't realized how much. He told me, but I had paid no attention. He didn't want his sheets or gown changed. It had been exhausting for him. Breathing was the priority. Damp gowns and sheets didn't matter at all. How could I have been so stupid? And the martini glass breaking was just the crowning blow . . . .

I sat there for several minutes trying to pull myself together. My gut instinct told me to go back to Sam's room and make peace with him, tell him again how sorry I was, how insensitive I had been, that I really cared about him. But I didn't go. I was afraid to. I went home instead.

That night I had no sleep. All I kept thinking about was Sam and his last words to me "Just go away." I had hurt and upset him terribly.

The next afternoon my husband and I left for a planned week-long trip to Toronto. I wanted to stop out to see Sam before we left, but was uncertain how he'd react after being so angry with me. Frankly, I was afraid to face him again, so I didn't go. We left on our trip.

I thought about Sam often over the five days away, thinking we'd reconcile when I returned home. I sent him a postcard from the King Edward Hotel promising to visit as soon as I returned.

On the road home I checked our voice mail on my cell phone. There was a message from Sarah saying Sam had died yesterday afternoon.

I cried.

Later that evening after we'd arrived home and unpacked, I searched the obituaries to see when and where the funeral for Sam would be. It was at 11 o'clock the next day.

At 10:30 the following morning I drove out to Hillside Cemetery, anxious to say my last "good-bye" to Sam.

The old wrought iron cemetery gates were wide open, but there were no cars around. It was empty and quiet. How odd, I thought. Usually there were workers here when there was a funeral, but there was no one in sight.

The maintenance facility was near the entrance so I drove over to it, jumped out of the car and knocked on the door. Shuffling sounds came from within. Finally the door opened and a caretaker appeared.

"I'm looking for Sam Wood's funeral, it's at 11 o'clock. There doesn't seem to be anyone here. Do you know where it is?"

"Oh, that one. Yeah, it was changed to 9:30 this morning so it's over. There were some relatives from out of town who had to get back so they moved it up earlier."

I was totally crushed. Now I'd missed the funeral too. I didn't even get to say good-bye to Sam. I got back in the car and drove out to Rose Arbor in search of Sarah. I really needed someone to talk to. Luckily, Sarah was in the nurses' break room catching up on her charts.

"Oh, Sarah, I'm so upset about Sam. I just missed his funeral. He got so angry at me the last time I saw him. He wasn't feeling good at all and I upset him terribly. He sent me away. He said, "Just go away." And I wanted to come see him the next day, but we went away. Now he's dead and I missed the funeral because the newspaper said it was at 11, but they changed it to 9:30. I feel just terrible. . . ." The words tumbled out as I started to cry.

Sarah got up from the table, came over to me and put her arm around my shoulders.

"Oh Anne, don't be so hard on yourself. You must feel awful that you missed his funeral. I know you and he had some special times together. Sam liked your coming to see him. Boy, he really loved having those martinis. We were all so amazed he was here this long. He took a drastic turn for the worse on Tuesday, and then got very bad the next day. But we've been expecting this for a while. Actually, Sam surprised us all by hanging on this long. Don't feel so bad. You were great for him. He adored you, you really perked him up."

Her words made me feel slightly better, but I regretted not having followed my gut instinct and having gone to see him after our "episode." At home I wrote Greg and his family a note, telling them how much I liked Sam and the hours we spent together and how sorry I was for their loss. I regretted not seeing Sam one last time. He drifted in and out of my thoughts for weeks afterwards.

~

Three months later towards the end of November I was standing in the supermarket deliberating over the lettuce when I heard a voice behind me say, "I know you—you're the martini lady."

It was Greg, Sam's son.

"Hello, Greg. How are you doing? I'm sorry I didn't get to your dad's funeral. I was out of town when he died. Sam was quite a guy."

"Anne, thank you for your nice note. Actually, we're doing OK. I've got to tell you, my dad really liked you—he just loved your coming to visit him, and talking with him and of course, bringing him his martinis. It was wonderful of you to do that for him. In case he never told you, I'm telling you now, he really appreciated it. So, thank you from all of us—you made his last days memorable, believe me."

I drove home that afternoon with my groceries, unpacked them and fixed myself a good-sized Glenfiddich on the rocks. I sat down in the living room in front of the fire and thought about Sam.

Our time together had been very special. He had loved his martinis in his special glass. In the months Sam had used the glass, I had thought to myself "What will I do with it when he's gone?" I could never let anyone else use it. It would always be *Sam's glass*. When it broke, I should have realized Sam was going to die soon. Sam had been breaking away slowly for the past four months and his final break was imminent. I had simply chosen to ignore it.

When I agreed to be Sam's volunteer, I was aware of his impending death. But as he and I spent those warm summer afternoons together drinking martinis and settling the problems of the world, we had forged a special friendship. I had become very fond of Sam and I didn't want to lose him.

Actually, Sam reminded me of my father whom I had absolutely adored. My father died twenty five years ago. I had not been there at his bedside, rather miles away when the call came in the middle of the night. I hadn't been able to minister to him in his last days either. I always regretted it. That feeling kept resurfacing during my months with Sam.

But I had been with my mother when she died in 1995. She and I loved each other deeply, but had had a tumultuous relationship over the years. The experience of being with her at the moment of death is one I will never forget, and I was able to care for her in her final days. Yes, that was what drew me to become a hospice volunteer. I sipped the scotch slowly and thought about the three of them: Daddy, Mother and Sam. They had all taught me different life lessons.

I miss them.

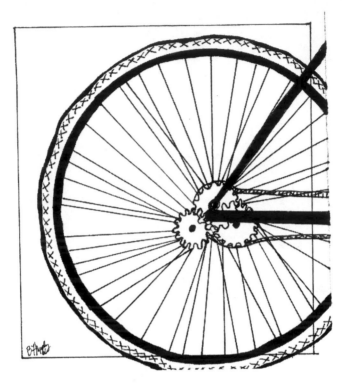

He Could Do No More
by Andrea Lanier

She seemed to stumble in drunken confusion across the Cologne Cathedral Plaza, but he knew she didn't drink. The incident was as brief as it was frightening, and repeated itself with cruel speed before all seemed normal again. A taxi returned them to their hotel where the concierge referred them to the nearest medical facility. The scan of Angela's brain showed a mass the size of a small cherry—a rare and radical brain-cell-attacking-and-eating tumor. In its efforts to encapsulate the tumor cells, Angela's brain tortured her with headaches.

Martin wanted to stay in Germany and have Angela treated immediately. Angela wanted to go home to see her children. By the time they arrived at the medical center back home, the tumor had doubled in size. The doctor marked a piece of paper with a tiny ink-dot. "One million cancer cells," he said. Martin was left to imagine how many would fit into the volume of two cherries. Life expectancy: six months. A desperate search for a more favorable prognosis failed. Six months of radiation and chemotherapy lay ahead of them but perhaps only to prolong her life for mere weeks.

I first welcomed Martin to my support group in early autumn 2003. His youthful shape disguised his age of late fifties. His demeanor was of gentleness and vulnerability. I sensed an uncommon combination of profound suffering and grace, with his humor not quite extinguished but severely traumatized. Martin's wife had just entered Rose Arbor Hospice. He had given up the fight of caring for her mostly on his own—"twenty-four/seven."

Martin was completely exhausted.

The sources of suffering and human response to pain and loss are infinite, but the universality of suffering in our lives provides a common thread that often unites us. A special kind of relationship developed between Martin and myself after his wife's death. It stemmed from his longing to be heard more deeply than the group setting allowed and my wish to understand better how people cope with terminal illness and what type of assistance might soften the impact of such trauma. I felt compelled to reach out to Martin. Not least, I hoped that our discussions might help relieve some of his grief and loneliness.

On Martin's invitation, one early morning in late October of 2003, I arrived at his historic home in the country. The scent of coffee brewing and Martin's melancholic smile greeted me as I walked through the door with the cinnamon coffeecake I'd just baked for the occasion. As always, when I can predict the answer, I am reluctant to ask, "How are you?'

"A beautiful home," I remarked.

"Too empty," Martin voiced what I'd sensed and went on: "I still talk to her—*Angela, I'm home!*—when I enter the house sometimes."

I didn't have to prompt Martin with questions. Sitting in the living room, next to a sunny window displaying colorful autumn foliage, he sought comfort from reminiscing just as naturally as he might quench his thirst at a fountain. "I was with her when she died," he began. "She was so beautiful. I met her when I was in Germany. She was working in the library on the Army base."

Listening to Martin, I had the privilege of hearing a beautiful love story that ended too tragically—too soon. With a gentle glow in his eyes, he reflected: "My entire life with her, thirty-six years, I was always afraid that someone would take her from me because she was so cool, so beautiful." Her picture on the fireplace mantle supported his description. He couldn't look, but limply moved his hand to indicate that I should. The picture showed Angela just before her death at fifty-nine, still attractive. Martin's memories transcended her glossy paper image. He could always see the stunning images of her youth— her laughter—her tears—her life— anytime he'd looked at her or thought of her, her aging a mere veil covering the timeless beauty of his love.

From the kitchen, I heard Martin's voice: "She was always so active. She did as much in fifty-nine years as another might in twice that many." But that had changed with the suddenness and violence of a brutal attack, an internal battle of brain cells against voracious cancer cells. The cancer ate away the encapsulation of Angela's brain. Within two weeks, she suffered a paralyzing stroke. Her bed was moved into the family room near a window that offered a view of a natural wildlife habitat—Martin knew this would please her. Ample shelves were lined with her books about theatre. Framed faces of her favorite theatre characters looked back at her from posters on the walls.

In the beginning, Martin was still able to assist her to the upstairs bathroom. She would lean into him and he would support her. But soon the cancer devoured Angela's speech, her vision, and her ability to write, to move.

"Marriage is work," Martin had said in the group. Angela had tried to mold him and refine him, make him love the theatre as she did and dress him in fine suits. She was frustrated with his long bicycling absences, yet they preserved their individuality in their relationship.

Sitting in his living room that day, Martin added that lately he was driven to seek a reprieve from his deepest pain by simply venting his anger. "She did this to me. . ." he mimicked with a spiteful voice what he'd say in his mind to escape his pain. But he also likened his spouse to "a nicely broken-in old shoe, so comfortable." And their marriage was of dancing, good conversation and laughter between the fights. He smiled mischievously. "But you know, from the beginning, we made wild and passionate love, frequently. The marriage could be in the toilet, but sex brought us back together every time. Argue, have sex, then make up."

When Martin spoke of Angela, his face often told much more than his words. Even his digression into anger could not disguise the deep sensuality of his love for Angela. His face shone with tenderness when he talked of their troubles, their fights, and their joys. While Angela was alive, Martin just tolerated the Broadway tunes she'd always play when they drove in her car. Now, since her death, he listened to her music.

Right after Angela's stroke, Martin cared for her in their home, bathing, feeding—providing anything and everything she needed. His family and several friends helped him so he could rest or leave the house for brief periods of respite. But soon the cancer devoured Angela's speech, her vision, and her ability to write and move. Martin had tried to do it all, but it was too painful and too tiring.

Finally, Martin called hospice. A nurse came out to see him, to evaluate Angela's condition and to help him set up a regular schedule for home hospice care. The hospice team was comprised of a doctor, nurse, home health care aid, chaplain, volunteer, and social worker. They were available as needed to monitor Angela's symptoms, adjust her medications, and bathe her. They also provided emotional support to Angela, Martin and their children.

Yet despite all the help, after two months, Martin was utterly fatigued.

"I did not want to get rid of her," he said. "I love her. But after two months into this thing, I realized that I couldn't do this anymore. Thirty radiation treatments and chemo—watching her slip away—she could no longer talk—she couldn't see—I could no longer move her—a friend of mine told me it was time, her quality of life had deteriorated completely. I let her be moved to Rose Arbor. I visited every day. The people there are very kind. It was not like a nursing home. There are a lot of volunteers, in addition to the staff. And a lot of times I would spend the night in the room with her. I'd wake up early, stay for another few hours, go home, and return again. In the morning, Angela would call out for me. But then I had to distance myself. I was becoming the husband again, and the Rose Arbor staff was becoming her caretaker. That was a blessing."

Martin's shoulders relaxed into his body, and the severity that had gripped his face disappeared as he relived the relief that he had felt when the hospice staff began to carry much of the load that had weighed him down.

Even before Angela died, Martin had found it difficult to make it through each day. When he came to my support group, he was relieved of some of his pain because he allowed the emotions he'd had to hold in most of the time come to the surface. He felt nurtured by the caring support of the other group members and appeared to take healing from offering his support to others. In group sessions, Martin evidenced a curious combination of courageously fighting his battles and graciously succumbing to his suffering.

But in the group, we did not hear about Martin's occasional screams of anguish. He said to me that he'd told no one else about those screams. He shouted them alone in his home in those moments when the "meteor of pain struck him viciously."

"Holy Mary, Mother of God," he'd shout. The words sustained him. He sought affirmation of his pain and received it.

"Angela wanted to come back home. She *did not* want to stay at Rose Arbor."

Then, he was compelled to say to her, "As much as I love you, I cannot…"

Her consequent disappointment pained him. Her disappointment translated into *his* thoughts as: *You should have done more—could have done more*—a relentless voice, but his own. He was filled with pain and guilt.

When Martin came to my group after his wife's move to Rose Arbor, I saw the exhausted man who could *not* have done any more. The affirmation from the group to this effect quieted his relentless voice of guilt only temporarily.

"I was with her when she died," he reflected. "The family, too. Her lungs were filling up with fluid. Her organs were shutting down. Then suddenly, it was like sitting in a room with someone I didn't know. I had no feelings. I felt relief. It was over. I felt numb. She'd suffered so much and never complained. Once I asked her what it was like. She said nothing. Her eyes filled with tears. And when I touched her face, she'd cried. If only I could have done more..." Martin wept.

I remember the first time he came to the group after her death—I could see it in his face. He told me he'd stood all night by the casket, composed. So many people came. So many expressed their condolences with cards, with flowers, and in person. But, suddenly, it all stopped.

"Then, I realized I was alone in this," Martin said. "That's when I knew I should have talked more with her. But she couldn't speak or write...One morning, I awoke feeling as if I were a mere hollow shell—I crashed, I yelled, I screamed—I stopped eating. No use feeding a hollow shell..."

For several weeks after Angela died, it seemed to Martin that his suffering was growing more intense. Martin has daughters and grandchildren for whom he wants to live and who bring light and joy into his life with visits, dinners, barbeques, and weekend trips. But even his love for his family can't overcome his loss.

Martin visited Angela's gravesite every day. "No one seems to understand," he said. "I even talk to her there, ask her how she's doing," he added, somewhat embarrassed.

Every day he struggled with the simplest tasks. He felt lost, paralyzed, robbed of mental and physical energy. Nevertheless, he forced himself to leave the huge, empty home he'd shared with Angela and go out each day. He visited the library and spent much time reading. He rode his bicycle with friends, one of whom sometimes accompanied him to the gravesite. His pastor came to visit Martin often. Martin continued visiting my group every week and the hospice grief counselor continued to see him regularly.

Before I left that day, I asked Martin what he wanted me to tell people about his experience and what did he want them to learn from him.

"Write that you mustn't lose hope. You must know that this is the worst thing you could ever go through. When other people tell you they know how you feel, they *do not*. And tell them, you *can't* snap out of it. You've got to work it out at your own speed. If people offer you help—*take it!*—even if you don't really believe you need it—or deserve it. If you are with a group of people, if you have episodes of tears coming, *expect* this to happen. Don't be afraid to let it happen. If people know you, they will understand. Don't hold it in. What you are going through is normal."

"Tell them to use anger wisely. It is a mechanism against feeling grief. Anger is expensive. You will dam up the feeling, and the anger stops the anguish—immediately. But you drop the anger and the grief will speed up. Sometimes you go numb. That's OK. If you were to go fully into grief, your personality would suffer. You must go in stages—repetitions—back up—forward. You do it incrementally. Have fun. Have guilt. Have anger. Feel sad. And you *will* have survivor guilt—*why not* *me?—she should live—*but then—she would suffer like I now do—she had always been afraid of that."

My talking with Martin confirmed for me that grieving traumatic losses remains inescapable. We cannot see that the words we didn't say or the things we failed to do would never have come to an end. We believe ourselves completely alone. We are convinced that no one could possibly understand our loss, our pain. Even when another person tells us of having endured identical circumstances, we still feel alone. We are convinced, *no one could possibly have endured what I'm enduring now and lived.*

In such times, the support net of love from family and friends has to catch us, carry us and sway with us in our internal storms without breaking, and teach us to trust our connections within that net. Frequently, even the most honestly expressed sympathy fails to penetrate and fill the painful void of aloneness generated by the loss of one held so dear. Yet, in our deepest aloneness, our faith in other people can help us cross the fragile bridges of similarities of human experience so that we might feel with each other to ease our suffering and pass through our grief.

Martin showed me the dimensions of his love, loss, vulnerability, his quiet courage, and his endless creativity to cope and survive. He showed me the external sources that cushioned his pain and eased his need to fight on his own. Along with Martin's family and friends, the staff of Rose Arbor Hospice played a most significant role, people he cherished because of their unique ability to care for him and his family and to understand their pain.

At the end of our conversation, escorting me outside via the garage, Martin showed me his beloved bicycle, a Trek 5900 Super-light road bike, silver and blue—top of the line. Without its chain and lock, it likely would have taken off even without its rider. We embraced by the door. He promised to call me if he needed to talk.

"You have to go visit Rose Arbor," he said to me as I walked away. "They hugged me when I was teary-eyed. They are my family."

"Yes, I will," I promised.

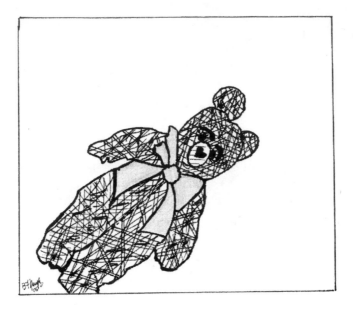

Teddy Bear
by Elizabeth Clark

Pollyanna smells like *Happy* perfume. She smells a lot like the kitchen. She's made from my Mommy's favorite robe.

Mommy liked to wear it when she'd make dinner. It got marynara and maccroni and cheeze (we call it M 'n' C) on it. It got little handprints from me and my brother tugging at her to get her to play with us. It got Playdoh and magic marker on it from our hands.

When Mommy died of breast cancer last year I was six and my little brother Chris was four. A nice lady made Mommy's robe into a teddy for me and a doggy for Chris. They're not like our other toys.

Daddy doesn't make us put Pollyanna and Colliash (that's Chris') in the toy-box when we clean up. They get to stay out and go to bed with us.

Sometimes I pretend Polly is Mommy and she tucks me in and tells me bedtime stories. Polly specially likes "Elmer the Elephant," 'cause it's got a rainbow elephant in it who gets in lots of silly trouble. Polly and Mommy and me all like rainbows. Polly's rainbow-ish like Mommy's robe was. It's a softy fabric Daddy calls "sheeneelle." She's one cozy friend.

Polly and Colly are made in "hug shape." Their arms and legs stick out to the side so you can just lean in and they hug you. I like that a lot.

When Mommy had to go to Rose Arbor, where you go when you're very, very sick, cozy robe went with her. We brought lots of things from home. We brought pictures of me and Chris and Daddy and Mommy having fun times at the park and at Christmas. We took her dangly guys that hang in our kitchen window that are made of magic stuff called led cristle (oops. . .Daddy said "lead crystal" is how that's spellt). Anyway, they make rainbows when it's sunny outside. Mommy would always swirl me around and say, "It's a rainbow day," when her danglies made rainbows on the walls. Sometimes she'd hold me up to the window and there was a rainbow on my cheek and she'd kiss my rainbow and tickle me under my chin. I really tickle there.

It was crummy Mommy not being at home. Mostly we stayed at the hospice place in a room across the hall. Sometimes Chris and me got to take a nap with Mommy in the afternoon when the rainbows came on her pretty quilty bedspread.

When Mommy wasn't feeling good, Chris and me sat at the table in the other room and made hearts for her out of our Playdohs. The table was special for us and had little chairs for us too.

I really miss Mommy. Sometimes I hug my Polly and cry and cry. Sometimes I see a red spot on Polly and wonder if it's from Mommy making us spaghetti. Chris doesn't have as many mom memories as me, but he still brings Colly everyplace with him.

Polly prefers playing Pretty, Pretty Princess. She lets me wear the tiaras because those dazzly sparkly things don't fit over her huge ears.

We feel sad for Daddy 'cause he doesn't have a Colly or Polly to cuddle, so we try to cuddle him extra lots. I know we're lucky that nice lady Mimi made our special friends for us. Daddy said a nurse lady from hospice told him about Mimi, the bear-maker.

I guess she makes softy friends for lots of kids like us who have mommies or daddies die, or grammys or popses, too. I guess robes and nightgowns make the best bears, because they're soft and smell just like the dead person you love who died.

Mimi makes them fast in only one day so you get your friend right away. I wish I knew how to make a bear. I would make one for Daddy, and one also for Mimi. She spends all her time working very hard. She tries to make kids like me and Chris feel better when their mom or dad dies. One time, I guess she made four bears even though she hurt her hand and had stitches and everything. That nice lady deserves a big hug. All the people at that Rose Arbor place were nice like that too. XOXO to you all. And XOXOXO also to Mommy up in heaven. I love you, Mommy. And I miss you.

The End

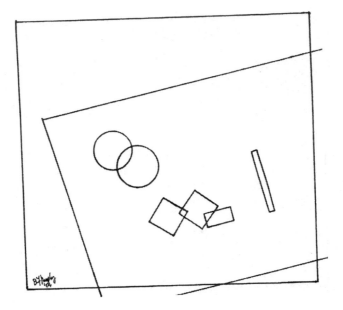

Less Is More
by Diana Fox

I never thought much about death as a young person. Since I had been married and divorced well before middle age, it never occurred to me that I needed a will. Nor did I ever think of myself as "dead," at least not until I became involved in the deaths of a dear friend, her husband, and my mother. Until that time, no one close to me had ever died. It was only in their deaths that I finally understood death, not only on a personal level, but also the logistics and implications to those left behind. As a result of those experiences, I became alive, and for the first time really began to live.

The first death that I experienced on an intimate level occurred suddenly. My friend, Judy, and I were in her kitchen. Her husband, Frank, came in from the yard where he'd been mowing the lawn and said he had to get more gas for the mower. He walked out to the garage, opened the car door and collapsed. The ambulance arrived quickly; Frank was resuscitated, but at the hospital Judy was told that as a result of the stroke, Frank was brain-dead. The next day, she and her two children made the decision to take Frank off all life-support machines. It wasn't a hard decision for the three of them to make because both Judy and Frank had the foresight to discuss not only what their death preferences were in such an emergency, but because they had documented their decisions legally and shared their choices with their children.

Watching Judy and her children dealing with Frank's death, I realized how negligent I'd been in tending to my own end-of-life affairs. I realized that if I were seriously injured, unable to communicate or, worse, died tomorrow, my son would suffer tremendously on multiple levels. He had no idea what my assets were, the location of paperwork he would need to contact insurances, banks, and firms with which I did business, or how I conducted my day-to-day affairs such as paying bills.

He also had no idea what my life preferences were in the event he should have to make a decision about my wanting to receive nutrition and water, water only, or nothing at all? If I were in a coma and he was told that I had brain activity, but no chance of living the same quality of life ever again, he had no way of knowing that my choice would be to die rather than be a burden to him or anyone. Judy's tragedy forced me to talk with my son regarding the care I wished to receive in the event of a catastrophic illness that left me incapable of making my own decisions. A Will and a Living Will both specified the procedures I wanted regarding my death. I soon had my preferences documented, filed them with my attorney, but more importantly, showed my son how to find everything he would need to act on my behalf. I showed him my files, where all my keys were, identified them for him, and we went over any other documentation he would need in order to handle my estate.

Before Frank's death, my friend Judy had been diagnosed with cancer. She had battled it bravely and won. Four years after Frank's death, however, she learned she needed further treatment, but the drug she needed only gave her a fifteen-percent survival rate. Fearing she wouldn't survive this round of treatment, I watched Judy pare her belongings and obligations down to the bare minimum. At first, her children and I protested. Eventually, we all gave in, realizing it was better for her health that we go along with her wishes.

Ken and Janet, her son and daughter, divided the antique furniture, photographs and other treasured artifacts of her life and ancestry. Judy's argument for giving clothing and other goods to her friends and charities now was that she would be saving her children time and heartache. She wasn't giving up. She simply was making life easier for her children in the event she didn't survive. It allowed her and everyone else the opportunity to talk about her illness and forthcoming death naturally. And in her own way, she got to tell everyone how much they each meant to her.

In the end, Judy had known best.

Less than a week after being told she needed another treatment, Judy entered Rose Arbor. Twelve days later, she died. It took her children only a few days to clean out her house and to settle her affairs. Judy would have liked that. She knew her children's own lives were complicated and consumed with work and family, and it was to that end that she sought to make her death easier for them. Because Judy had been so open about death, encouraging everyone around her to talk about it, those she loved and left behind were able to mourn her passing respectfully but with little stress. Even in death, Judy had been more concerned about the living.

Then came my most difficult experience in dealing with death: my mother died. In retrospect, I know now it was the most difficult only because it was the longest. I also know had I not experienced Frank's and Judy's deaths, I would not have been able to cope well with Mother's illness—let alone her death. Their deaths had made me strong. I would need to call upon that strength time after time.

Mother had broken her hip a few years before and while recuperating, was forced to live with me. But after her recovery, she chose to return to her own apartment where she lived alone. Mother wasn't a big woman, but after she recovered from her broken hip, she became even more frail. When I finally convinced her to see a doctor again, we learned she had lung cancer. The disease didn't hamper her desire for independence and determination to live alone. She wanted to maintain her own home as long as possible.

I saw that this wasn't going to be possible, but it took a number of discussions and the help of health experts to convince Mother that she needed the help of hospice. It was Judy who had educated me about hospice and Rose Arbor. When Mother finally agreed to move to Rose Arbor, it was only with the promise that I would keep her apartment intact. Her greatest fear was that she would recover but have no home. I knew Rose Arbor would be her last residence, but I kept that insight to myself.

The average life expectancy of Rose Arbor patients is three months. As we approached that anniversary mark, I worried. Would we be kicked out? I need not have worried. The staff let me know that Mother's comfort was of foremost importance, no matter the length of time it took either to return her to health and go home, or to die there. Occasionally, there were residents who *did* recover from a life-threatening illness and were well enough to leave Rose Arbor. Because Mother anticipated going home, and because she was a stubborn woman who refused to talk about difficult subjects, including death, money and her own affairs, I was never able to have the conversations I needed to have with her. Anytime I tried to broach one of these topics, she quickly changed the subject.

Because Mother would never talk about any of this, I began to wander about the halls of Rose Arbor. I'd hear snippets of conversations, see residents and their families in varying degrees of comfort or distress. Residents came and died, with new residents moving in. Soon, I realized that for every resident room in Rose Arbor, there was a different story.

Then, three months after arriving at Rose Arbor, Mother died. When one of the volunteers asked if there was anything she could do for me, I said, "Play tennis for me tonight." The surprised look on her face suggested it wasn't the response she had expected, but I knew I wouldn't be able to play in my league, so I was concerned about finding a substitute. One truth Judy had taught me was that life goes on. It is best not to brush it aside, because it is in living that one heals. I witnessed Judy practice that truth when Frank died; she was right.

Ironically, trying to settle Mother's affairs became more stressful than her actual death, but finally her estate was in order. Throughout the ordeal, I thought often about my own life and realized I was cheating myself and those I loved. As a result, I simplified my life, adopting Judy's motto of "Less is more." With fewer possessions to protect or maintain, I find myself spending more time with people, with books, and studying in greater depth the experience of death. Actually, I had been more afraid of watching someone close to me die rather than death itself. Now I find deep pleasure in the minute details of every day life. Best of all, I no longer fear death.

Less is More

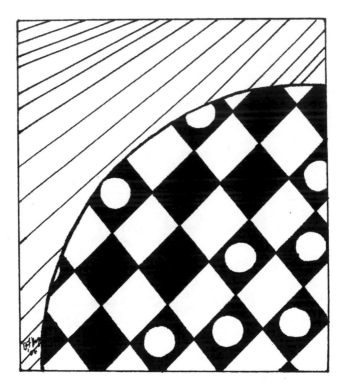

Win by Losing
by Beth Carroll Van Houten

Jim was seventy-four when he met George, a volunteer with Hospice. By this time Jim had had multiple strokes and received hospice care at home. Because of the strokes, he had lost most of the control of his mouth, including the ability to speak, swallow, and control his saliva, which dripped on a bib he wore. He had also lost most of the feeling in his hands, but he was still able to walk.

Jim's house was a medium-sized ranch home painted creamy tan with brown shingles. The large yard was covered in deep green grass with a small rose garden, and was edged with a "forest" of white pine trees on one side. George later learned that Jim and his wife had built their home. They had the true pioneering spirit. Jim's wife, Lois, had done much of the plumbing and all of the wallpapering.

George's first visit with Jim was troubling. When Lois opened the door to welcome him, George could see the tears in her eyes and faintly hear Jim's whimpering in the next room. She led George into the kitchen to Jim before she returned to her chores. Jim cried throughout George's visit, making it difficult for George to learn much about him. Lois puttered about the house in a daze, trying not to let tears mirror her husband's emotions.

This scenario continued on the next two visits. George spent these visits wondering how to lift Jim's spirits. As a hospice volunteer, he was supposed to be a friend to the patient during the end of his life, but he found it difficult when Jim was almost always crying. It was visibly difficult on his friends and family to see their husband, father, grandfather—a World War II veteran—so distraught by his situation in life, and there was nothing they could do to help him. George realized how Jim's tears were affecting his family, so being the straightforward, blunt man that he was, he had a talk with Jim during his third weekly visit.

"Jim, you're a World War II vet; being in that war, you showed a lot of courage, courage to get through the day and get through the war until you came home," George said. "Were you scared in the war?"

Jim replied in nods and shakes of his head, and sometimes with hand gestures. Jim nodded a "yes."

"Are you scared to die?"

Jim nodded again.

"You had courage in the war. Now you should try to overcome your fear of death with that same courage," George continued. "Your family and friends love you very much, and it hurts them to see you upset all the time. They are sad about your condition, but want to make the best of the time they have with you. Now, why don't you demonstrate that courage again by not crying and try to be a little more cheerful?"

Jim let the thought sink in; his tears slowed down some.

"I'm gonna let you think on that—I need to head home. I'll see you next Tuesday, as usual. Have a good week, Jim," George said as he stood up to leave. "You're a strong man, and a good fellow. 'Til next week."   And with a nod of his head, George left.

When he returned the following week, he was surprised to learn from Lois that Jim had hardly cried since he had left the week before. Jim didn't cry from then on during George's visits. He even smiled on occasion. Not surprisingly, this had a positive affect on everyone who came in contact with Jim. It caused Lois to pick up. She began talking to George about their past: falling in love as childhood sweethearts, Jim's business, and family stories. Then one day she told George about Jim's reputation at checkers.

"You know," Lois said, "Jim loves to play checkers. It's his game—nobody can beat him."

George looked at Jim, seeing a rare smile and a sparkle in his eye. "That true Jim?"

Jim smiled more broadly and with a shrug that said "Find out," opened his eyes wide.

"How 'bout a game, Jim?" George asked.

With a smile and a nod from Jim, Lois got the checker board out of the closet and handed it to George. The men walked from the kitchen into the living room. Jim sat on the cushiony couch, facing

George who sat on an oak chair he carried in from the kitchen. They faced each other over the coffee table where George set up the red and black plastic pieces on the laminated cardboard playing board. With a rub of his palms, Jim moved a black checker, and the game began. George moved a red one. Back and forth they went, turn by turn, the pieces coming off the board one by one. When an opportunity came for George to jump three of Jim's men, without thinking George took the three pieces, tying up the game by leaving two kings for each man.

"It's a draw," George said.

Jim answered with a strong shake of his head. He seemed to yell 'NO!' with this simple movement. Jim stared intently at the board. George became concerned that the game would cause Jim to have another stroke, but they continued to move pieces. George kept his pieces from being caught until he purposely moved a piece to where Jim could jump it and take the game. Jim smiled victoriously.

"You won! Well, you live up to your reputation!" George told Jim. "I've been beaten!" The men sat together until it was time for George to leave.

As George drove home that afternoon, he thought about the checker game. Why had he been so competitive in a board game against a dying man? Against a man who didn't have much longer to live—what did he have to gain? He suddenly understood what he needed to do. By letting Jim win, they both left the game winners—it made them both feel happy, as if they had accomplished something. Checkers was Jim's game; this was one of the last ways he could keep his self esteem, keep his control. George realized that winning a game is not important—making others happy and serving others in anyway he could, this what winning was for him.

Over the next two months during their visits together, Jim never brought out the checkerboard again. George never knew whether it was because Jim thought George let him win or because the game was so close at the end.

George would take Jim for rides, which both men enjoyed. George would drive around town, talking to Jim about some of his favorite places and restaurants. Jim would communicate to George through pointing and making small groaning sounds, as they passed Jim's favorite restaurant, Sicily's Best, a local Italian place known for its spaghetti and meatballs. Jim would point and tap on the window when they rode past the red and green striped awning, push his lips together and say, "mmmmmmmm" and rub his stomach in the circular 'yumm' motion.

Sometimes the two men would play cribbage. George would win a cribbage game once in a while to keep the games interesting. When Jim moved the pegs on the scoreboard, there were times he would move too far because he did not have much control or feeling in his hands. At first, this upset George— it was like Jim was cheating! He reminded himself whom he was playing against and that, either way, win or lose, he would win.

During one visit, they played three games of cribbage. Jim won all three games, intensely proud of his accomplishment. As George left that day, Lois asked how many games they had played and who won. Jim held up three fingers and pointed proudly at his chest with a big smile. George felt the same way about himself—a victorious winner in a losing game.

After George left that late summer day, Jim climbed onto his riding lawn mower and drove the perimeter of his property. As Lois watched him, she could see he seemed proud of his life. Later she told George about what she saw her husband do on his drive. He drove past the blossoming roses that were beginning to wilt. He stopped the mower long enough to climb off and smell his favorite white rose. Lois continued to watch Jim as he glanced into the "forest."

She began thinking of how their family had grown like a forest, beginning with a few trees and seeds—the two of them--and expanding into a forest of a family with children and grandchildren and sons and daughters-in-law. He rode to the edge of their property, and gazed over the hill and up into the sun that was peeking from behind a cloud. He closed his eyes and tilted his head up, feeling the warmth of the sun on his face, seeing the warmth in hues of red, orange and yellow from under his eyelids. As she watched him, Lois prayed that Jim was content.

Later that same day, Jim's condition changed suddenly. He was taken quickly to Rose Arbor where he stayed for only one night. He passed away quietly the next day.

George attended Jim's funeral. There he noticed that Jim was dressed the way he lived, honestly and unpretentiously, in a wool plaid sport shirt. Jim's son-in-law spoke at the service. "Jim never had much in life financially, but he was always looking out for you, looking to help others, whether it was trying to find someone a better job or helping them become a better person," the son-in-law said. "He welcomed me into the family as his own son when I married his youngest daughter. He always asked if we needed anything—anything at all— whether it was money for a down payment on a car, or help building a shed, he was always there. He listened to problems, but only offered advice if asked. He was unselfish, a truly giving person."

And that is a large part of winning by losing, George thought. Truly winning is a selfless act of giving, not wanting to receive anything in return. You cannot help others without receiving something in turn; a better attitude, a new lease on life, or just the sense of knowing you have done well. Givers always win. And Jim and George were winners.

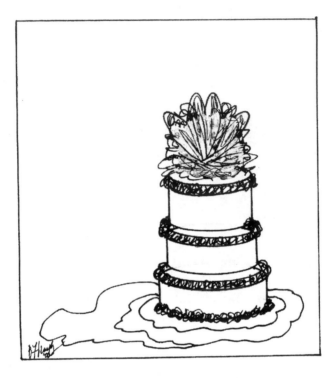

The Wedding
by Matthew Crowe

When Dr. Burns diagnosed her cancer, he told Charlotte to expect six more months, maybe eight with good fortune. Nine months later she returned to his office for a checkup, and teased him about living on borrowed time.

"I've always been an over-achiever," she told him with a wink. "You know I can't leave before my grandson gets married. After that, I'll think about leaving."

"I should've known," he replied smiling softly, gently shaking his head. "I could tell you were feisty, but I just didn't realize how strong you were."

But two weeks later, Charlotte no longer felt feisty or strong. Her appetite had all but disappeared, and her eighty-plus years old frame was becoming thinner and frailer with each passing day. She spent more and more time sleeping, and her four daughters were taking turns staying at her home to watch over her. They also arranged for hospice to come in.

By mid-January, her daughters were exhausted by the late nights and irregular schedules. It was then that her oldest daughter Jackie introduced the idea of moving their mother to Rose Arbor. "A woman from church volunteers there, and she's always had nothing but wonderful things to say about the place. I went there today, and I think she was right. It doesn't feel like a hospital, but there are nurses around all the time. I think it might be good for mom. For us too."

Her sisters were reluctant to agree. They didn't want to quit on their mother, but they agreed to visit Rose Arbor to see for themselves. Two days later, after speaking to the program director and walking through the halls, the sisters all conceded that Rose Arbor really seemed right for their mother.

Four days later, Jackie helped her mother settle into her new room at Rose Arbor. She brought a duffel bag with clothes and some personal items, and she also brought a brown paper bag filled with pictures of Charlotte's children, grandchildren and great grandchildren. Charlotte had spent the past five years as a widow after sixty years of marriage, and always said she was happiest around her family. Now their framed faces surrounded her bed, resting on tables, windowsills and the top of her television set. On the table to the left of her bed sat an engagement picture of Jackie's oldest son, John, and his fiancée, Mary.

Their wedding was in two weeks, and Jackie, who was an ordained minister, was going to conduct the ceremony in the family church downtown. As she lay on her pillow, Charlotte gazed at the picture with tired eyes. She knew she wouldn't be able to attend; her stamina was simply too low. The thought of traveling to the church was overwhelming, and she didn't want her presence to burden anyone. She insisted that John and Mary carry on with their wedding as planned, and not worry about her. She promised to see the pictures as soon as they were developed, and she honestly wouldn't mind resting alone for a day.

Jackie had watched her mother's health decline during the past three weeks, and she feared she wouldn't live to see the wedding. She tried coaxing Charlotte into attending, but deep down she knew her mother wouldn't be able to leave Rose Arbor. Jackie also knew that behind the brave façade, Charlotte wanted more than anything to see her grandson get married.

With little other recourse, Jackie, John and Mary met with the director of Rose Arbor and asked if there was any possibility that they could have the wedding on the premises at Rose Arbor. "The guest list is small, and the Great Room down the hall would fit all of us comfortably. We'd like to include the other patients and staff too." Although no one had ever considered having a wedding at Rose Arbor, the director and staff all agreed it was a wonderful idea.

After the meeting, John and Mary went to their grandmother, Charlotte, with their decision. The two sat next to the bed holding hands, and John told her the news. Charlotte covered her mouth in surprise, and tears welled in her eyes. Without speaking, she motioned them both to her bed and she hugged them together and whispered into their ears, "Thank you. Thank you so much."

When John and Mary left to go home, Charlotte sat up and talked to Jackie about the new wedding plans, and spoke with more energy than she had in the past month. The ceremony was to take place in seven days, and until that day Charlotte spoke of little else. She talked about which dress she might wear, and about who was going to attend and where everyone would sit during the ceremony. Every time her daughters came to visit, they would push Charlotte in a wheelchair and sit in the Great Room to talk about the wedding plans.

The wedding took place on a Saturday afternoon in late February. That morning, Charlotte's granddaughters, Claire and Robin, came to help her get ready. Claire brought a red dress from Charlotte's house, and Robin helped her put makeup on for the ceremony. Charlotte hadn't worn makeup in months, and she felt happy to dress up again. With Robin dabbing blue eye shadow on her closed lids and Claire painting her nails red, Charlotte joked: "I feel like I am getting ready for the prom."

By the time they left her room to go down the hall, Charlotte's gray hair was perfectly braided, and with makeup on she looked healthier than she had in months. Her favorite pearl necklace hung around her neck, cascading over her high collar. Below her left shoulder she wore a white rose, just like the one John wore on the lapel of his black tuxedo.

Heavy snow had fallen the night before, and the wind drifted powder against the icy edges of the Great Room windows. Through the window the ground radiated electric white, illuminating the makeshift chapel. The room's usual tables and couches were moved to the side and placed in front of the bookshelves. In their place were five rows of dark, weathered-oak folding chairs with thin, black leather padded seats. An aisle split the chairs into two equal sections of five rows, and small bouquets of red and white roses were tied with ribbons onto the backs of the chairs on the inside aisle.

When the ceremony was about to begin, John guided Charlotte's wheelchair to her place in the front row, and he kissed her on the cheek before turning to join his mother, who was the minister, waiting for them at the altar. When Mary appeared in the doorway, everyone rose and turned to see her walk softly in her snow white dress. Jackie held her black leather Bible across her chest, and John stood with his hands clasped together. When Mary came near, John offered his hand and drew her close to his side. While they stood together exchanging their vows, Charlotte sat quietly, smiling and occasionally dabbing her eyes with a white handkerchief. She was careful not to let her tears smear her makeup.

After the ceremony, a small reception was held in the back of the room. Everyone mingled quietly for about an hour, and Charlotte ate half a piece of marble wedding cake. She raved about the frosting.

Eventually, the guests all said their goodbyes and filed out the door. John, Mary and Jackie stayed to help Charlotte back to her room and into bed. She was obviously exhausted, so the newlyweds quickly hugged her and said goodbye.

As the setting sun filled the room with soft red light, Jackie sat alone near Charlotte's bed and waited for her mother to fall asleep. When she decided to go, she softly held her mother's hand to tell her goodbye, and then left her alone to rest. It had been a wonderful day. Charlotte slept peacefully through the night.

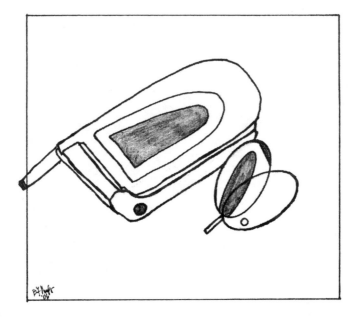

Twenty-Six Hours
by William Zinkus

By 2:00 p.m. Wednesday the ambulance has delivered her safely to Rose Arbor. Her family arrives shortly thereafter, a tired, haggard-looking threesome of father, daughter and son. They walk through the entranceway and are greeted by a nurse, who tells them where to find Mother.

The room is down at the end of the wing. The family shuffles past open doors on either side of the hallway, and the son remarks to his sister that he finds the silence both comforting and eerie. They see no visitors in the rooms they pass, only the occasional patient asleep in bed or propped up in a chair watching television. The daughter whispers that she feels funny about looking too closely into the rooms, as if she is invading someone's privacy, even though the curiosity is natural and honest.

The husband has said nothing so far. He appears the weariest of the three, but considering his age—he'll turn eighty-seven in a couple weeks—and considering that he, too, had been recently hospitalized for a heart condition, he looks relatively fit. Someone from the Rose Arbor staff asks if he would like to sit down for a moment, for

Room 12 is still a goodly distance away. He smiles and says no thanks, if he can't make it that far without resting, then maybe they should prepare a room for him!

The family approaches Room 12 together, walking side-by-side, and there is an awkward moment by the doorway when no one wants to be the first to go inside. After an instant's hesitation the son breaks free and steps through the door. Close behind follows the daughter, and finally the husband, who comments on the fine carpentry of the ceiling and the pleasing October afternoon light that pours through the windows and skylight. He says the room is larger than he expected, and cheerier, in a way. Then he spots the couch at the other side of the room and the son immediately knows what his father is thinking: a nap. And there the father goes, but first he must pass where his wife of sixty years lies, comatose, unresponsive since the morning five days before when he found her.

The daughter and the son move away from the bed. The two nurses who had been settling Mother in have disappeared. None of the family remembers their leaving the room. The father cautiously comes to the side of his wife, hoping for a sign that she might be aware of his presence. Her breathing is difficult and uneven and shallow, aided by an oxygen line that snakes away toward a whirring, humming machine in the bathroom. He makes a mental note to ask someone if there is a way to make the machine quieter, or to possibly shut the bathroom door to mute the constant drone. But as quickly as he thinks to do this, he forgets. Instead he takes his wife's hand in his and strokes her pallid smooth skin with a gentleness and a calm that neither of the two children has seen in their father before.

~

The family has names, of course: the husband is Vince; the daughter, Adrienne; the son, Adrienne's younger brother, is Daniel; and the mother is Shelley, although Vince always calls her Mommy in the presence of their children, a habit he never lost from the days long ago when they all were young and a habit that now seems unbearably sad. Another brother, an older one named Patrick, lives in Memphis.

Only a few days before Daniel had been sitting next to his mother on the sofa at home, helping her work the New York Times crossword puzzle. Adrienne sat across the living room in the new chair, telling a long story about her cats that nobody seemed to be listening to. He remembers how his mother asked for a four-letter word meaning "crazy"—he suggested "daft"—and then a few minutes later asked for a seven-letter word for "rifle" beginning with "C." Before he could even respond, she said it must be "carbine," and it was. Everything was so normal that afternoon. The day before his mother had finished the last of her chemotherapy treatments and she was actually looking forward to a solid meal that night. She had been a bit confused that morning—she poured oatmeal into the coffee maker instead of coffee grounds, and thought the day was Sunday instead of Friday—but the facility with which she worked the crossword puzzle and the excitement she voiced at the prospect of seeing her two new great-grandchildren later in the month made the morning lapse seem fleeting and insignificant and almost comical.

The next morning—a Saturday—Daniel came back from a long walk to find his answering machine flashing in what he will always recall as a frantic manner. The first message, left an hour before, was from his dad: Mommy was in trouble, and could he get over to the house as soon as possible? Please? The second message, time-stamped fifteen minutes later, was from his sister-in-law, in Tennessee: did he know that Mom was in the emergency room at the hospital? Adrienne had called him several times but there was no answer. Apparently, too, his cell phone was turned off. You'd better get down to the hospital, Daniel!

~

Only an hour later visitors arrive at Room 12: more relatives and friends. Now the hospice room is full and vital with activity. Vince sits at the table by the window, talking about golf with their neighbors, the Robinsons. Two cousins are watching cable news on the small TV while Adrienne sips coffee. Daniel is nowhere to be seen as he has gone home to take a shower and change his clothes.

But on the way Daniel has stopped by the office to talk with a hospice nurse named Ruth, who turns out to be the cousin of one of his closest high school buddies.

Somehow, after a conversation of only three minutes, Daniel knows that Ruth, the nurse responsible for taking care of his mom during the day shift, is one of the most remarkable persons he has ever met. She has a serene way about her, a soothing voice, an air of compassion so genuine that he cannot imagine how she can go about her daily work without using herself up. She looks him straight in the eye as she explains that his mother may not even last through the night, that his sister and father or whomever plans to stay this evening should pay close attention to her breathing patterns because there are certain unmistakable signs. She gives Daniel a thin booklet with a summary of what she has told him and says he shouldn't worry about going home to clean up, but on the other hand he shouldn't dilly-dally, either.

~

Daniel has not slept more than a couple of hours at a time for nearly a week, and he feels sluggish and stupid in the head. Those five days and four nights at the hospital wore him down. There were endless probings and blood draws and diagnostic tests performed on his mother. He watched a conveyor belt of doctors, nurses, technicians, orderlies, machines, carts, trays, and gurneys flow into and out of her room in the ER—and finally, after a day and a night of speculation, a neurologist brought the family together and told them that Shelley had suffered a profound brain seizure, brought on by encephalitis. The neurologist showed them the MRI picture of her brain, which had suffered massive damage, and said there was a less than ten percent chance of her regaining consciousness. Even then, the doctor added, and assuming she could eventually be taken off the respirator, Shelley would be incapable of moving or talking or caring for herself in any way.

You have a decision to make, the doctor said, looking directly at Vince but speaking to all of them. Why don't you sleep on it, and we'll talk again tomorrow morning?

Daniel and his sister and his father spent the night discussing the situation. Everyone agreed that being kept alive by a machine was no way to live. Mommy told me many times to just let her go if that ever happened, said Vince again and again.

So the next morning they asked the doctor to let her go. There would remain an oxygen mask to help her breathe on her own, and plenty of medication for any pain that she might be feeling. She would stay in the ICU until she stabilized. She might last a day or many weeks.

But when the meeting with the doctor was near conclusion, Vince began to have sharp chest pains and trouble breathing. Adrienne rushed to the nursing station and five minutes later Vince was in an examination room in ER, soon to be admitted to the coronary unit for overnight observation and monitoring.

~

Daniel returns to Rose Arbor around dinner time. On the table in Room 12 are three meals, one each for him and Adrienne and their father. Everyone else has left. Then Adrienne decides now would be a good time to run home, feed the cats and get cleaned up herself. She volunteers to come back and stay the night, this first night, and then perhaps they all could take turns afterwards? From the moment Vince found his wife the previous Saturday morning, she has not been alone, and without actually saying so, the family vows that she will never be alone, regardless how long she stays at the hospice.

During the meal Vince says again how pleasant the room is, that they made the right choice to move Mommy here instead of watching her die in the sterile hospital room. She would like it here, he says, his voice softening and then trailing off to near inaudibility. Daniel can think of nothing to say in response. He nods his head and reaches for his father's hand. The only sound in Room 12 is the muted humming from the bathroom, and of course the gasping, rattling sound of Mommy struggling for her breath.

~

That second night in the hospital consisted of Daniel pushing his father back and forth in a wheelchair, from the coronary unit to ICU.

Adrienne and Daniel agreed: the hospital was the best place for Dad to be. That night Daniel would sleep in the ICU room with their mother until 2 a.m., then Adrienne would spell him. Their father was given a sleeping pill around 11 p.m., and would not awaken before breakfast time.

~

Adrienne is back with an armful of pillows and a comforter and some puzzle books. One of the nurses from the evening shift—the family never does catch her name—is taking vital signs and adjusting the flow of oxygen and telling them Shelley may need another pain med. Daniel makes his living teaching English at the university but has never really thought about the meaning of the word "palliative" before. Earlier he noticed a dictionary in the Great Room library; he walks down there and reminds himself that "palliative" means easing the pain of a disease, but not effecting a cure.

Daniel's cell phone alerts him to an incoming call. His brother Patrick wonders what is going on—why haven't they kept him informed? Too quickly Daniel replies: You said before to call if there's any change. There hasn't been any change.

Well, let me know if there is, okay?

Pat, the only change will be when Mom dies.

Silence. Uncomfortable silence.

Let me know.

I will.

~

Less than six hours have passed.

The brilliant autumn day ends in a blaze of reds and yellows hanging close above the western horizon. There is no change in Shelley.

Room 12 takes on a somber cast as the evening light wanes through shades of diluted orange, umber and, finally, a dull gray liquid dusk settles over the room. Daniel tries to make small talk with his cousins, neither of whom he's felt particularly close to over the years, but he cannot concentrate on anything they are saying. His mind conjures a slide show of scenes of growing up, images of joy and heartbreak, pleasure and pain, fulfillment and longing -- all these become more real than the conversation itself. He sees a warm night during one long summer at the Lake Michigan cottage, the summer after their youngest brother died in

Colorado and indelibly, his mother and father watching another glorious sunset with tears in their eyes. It's just so goddamned beautiful his mother says, when he asks her if she's all right. His father nods in agreement. He leaves them alone on the deck of the cottage. He sees the money tree the whole family chipped in for as a present on her fiftieth birthday: fifty crisp one dollar bills attached to the branches of a spindly evergreen of some sort or the other. Then, in rapid succession, his mother's look of pride, the afternoon she came home after making a hole-in-one at the St. Joe Valley golf course; her concentration when she ironed freshly laundered shirts, something she claimed to actually enjoy; her weariness on the last day of the chemotherapy cycles; a few days later, delight at the baby-sized chocolate-almond ice cream cone from Dean's dairy in Plainwell.

Daniel is staring now, just over the shoulder of his Uncle John, where Mommy lies peacefully in the hospice bed. Every now and then she seems to be panting, gasping for air, but the effect lasts only a moment and her respirations return to a ragged, shallow regularity. A nurse slips into the room and checks the vital signs, adjusts the oxygen mask, tells them all that it's time to turn Shelley and freshen the bedclothes. Daniel smiles at the mention of the word 'bedclothes,' so disconnectedly old-fashioned is the word, but so comfortable, too. Everyone leaves the room while the nurse and the aide perform their duties.

The nurse and the aide are finished. They find Daniel standing alone in the hall outside the door to Room 12. Adrienne has left to walk the Robinsons to their car, and cousins are with Vince down in the Great Room. The nurse tells Daniel he can go back in now.

His mother lies as before, but now, clean and refreshed and propped up on her left side with a pillow. She almost looks comfortable. There are two small teddy bears—one bear holding the other—in her arms. The old purple, glass-bead rosary is arranged in her hands, the sixth 'Hail Mary' of the fourth decade between her thumb and forefinger. The faint scent of lotion clings to her as Daniel leans close to kiss her forehead. He wonders if she knows anything, if she can hear or feel or sense anything at all. Once, a few days before in the hospital, Daniel ran his fingernail up the arch of her foot, and he knows he saw her twitch in response.

But since then, there has been no sign whatsoever.

Daniel takes his father home for the night, then, at the old man's urging, heads home to sleep in his own bed for a change.

Surprisingly, everyone—even Adrienne, who spends the night in Room 12 on the pull-out bed—everyone gets a good night's rest. A weight has been lifted, or so goes the cliché, and in the morning over breakfast—Daniel and his father bring bagels and fruit and piping hot coffee—they reaffirm the good sense of the decision to move her from the hospital to Rose Arbor. . .only the day before? The eighteen hours since the transfer have crawled by in slow suspension.

~

The ICU manager had come in early in the morning to inform them that Shelley would have to be moved to a regular room now that she had stabilized. Trouble was, there were no rooms available, and the hospital desperately needed the ICU bed. There were several options to be considered: first, a temporary holding room in ER, while they waited for a regular room to open up; second, a long-term care facility. Why don't you just say nursing home? Daniel thought with irritation at the time. Because there's no way of knowing how long your mother will. . .the manager's voice trailed off as she searched for another way to say, how long your mother will live. And third, in fifteen minutes or so the hospital social worker would talk to them about another possibility. The ICU manager left it at that.

The other possibility, of course, was taking Mother to Rose Arbor, if they had a room available. There are only eighteen rooms in all, but there's a fairly good turnover, the social worker said, then caught himself and apologized for the phrasing. You know what I mean, don't you? he asked. The four of them were having the conversation in a claustrophobic conference room just off the corridor to the ICU. The air in the room was close, and the walls bore prints and paintings that were supposed to be pleasing to the eye. I'll leave you these brochures, the social worker said—he was a rotund, soft, aging man, not the young and pretty and compassionate woman Vincent had spoken to for a moment the evening before—and you can think about what you want to do with Mother.

I wish he'd stop calling her Mother, Adrienne said, after he left them alone. She's not his mother.

~

Around eleven Adrienne asks Daniel if he minds staying alone with Mom for an hour or so, while she runs a couple of errands and takes Dad for a haircut. Then you can go over to school when I get back, she says, or wherever it is that you said you had to be this afternoon.

Room 12 basks in the warm and sunny afternoon. Daniel opens a couple of windows after everyone is gone. Faintly, from somewhere, comes the muted thrashing, grinding sound of a mower, but otherwise the day is peacefully uneventful.

Daniel suddenly feels drowsy; he arranges the cushions from the sleeper couch on the floor and gingerly lies down. His back has been giving him a hard time. At the beginning of the summer he learned that one of the discs in his lower back had a bulge, a herniation, that was pressing against the sciatic nerve and sending shooting pains down his left leg. Ruefully, he recalls the way he spent his summer—flat on his back, mostly, reading a new book every couple of days—and every afternoon driving over to see Mom, who invariably was resting on the sofa, watching "M*A*S*H" or working a crossword. One time, when Daniel burst into tears at his mother's discomfort, she motioned him over and held him close until he stopped weeping. He knelt beside the sofa with his head to her chest, his folks' old dying golden retriever

Oliver licking the side of his face and nuzzling his hand for some scratching behind the ears.

But just as Daniel begins to drift off to sleep —with the help of a Vicodin that his doctor has prescribed for just such an occasion—he hears activity in the room and sees Ruth and a helper at his mother's bedside. The time is 2 p.m., just twenty-four hours since the admission to Rose Arbor. Ruth is fluffing pillows and the helper is smoothing lotion into his mother's parched skin.

When Ruth is finished with her task she signals Daniel to follow her out to the hall. Your mother's breathing has changed, she says calmly, but the gravity of the news is unmistakable. Where are your dad and your sister?

Daniel notices that three hours have passed since Adrienne left. Should I call them? he asks Ruth.

You should, Ruth replies, and takes his hand in hers. It is very close, she says in a gentle, low voice.

Adrienne is on her way, stuck in traffic on Drake Road near the new university engineering campus.

Again, Daniel is alone with his mother in Room 12. There is liquid portent in the air, a palpable, foreboding sense of change that he has not felt before this. But oddly enough, now his mother's breathing seems to come more easily, and whether indeed a fact or born of wishful thinking, she looks at peace, with a hint of a smile on her lips.

Adrienne and Vincent come rushing into the room ten minutes later.

Adrienne wants to speak to Daniel alone. Vincent sits down beside Mother and holds her hand. The siblings walk down the hall toward the Great Room, then step through the double door to the patio. The sun is very warm and the day is still. I don't think she's going to last much longer, Adrienne says.

That's what Ruth thinks, too.

I was so worried Mom would die while I was gone. Adrienne sniffs back her tears, and Daniel puts his arm around his sister.

We can't all be there twenty-four hours a day. You've been with her constantly, Adrienne. Nobody's done more than you have. If you're not there—if I'm not there, or Dad's not there—we can't feel guilty about it.

I know.

Just keep your phone handy. I'll call, or you call, but one of us should always be with Dad. If we have to take a break, then we just have to.

They walk back to Room 12, holding hands. Vincent is still sitting beside the bed. Adrienne turns on the TV and settles on a show where the audience is screaming at a smug young man on stage who claims not to be the father of a fat woman's child.

Daniel cannot stand it. He tells everyone he's going for a walk. But first he goes over to the bed, kisses his mother's forehead, straightens the teddy bears and, as an afterthought, advances the purple rosary beads in her clenched hand to the fifth decade.

Halfway to the lobby Daniel encounters Dr. Brown, the hospice staff physician. I was just going in to see your mom, the doctor tells him.

My dad's in there with my sister, is all Vincent can think to say. Maybe I'll wait here until you're finished?

Five minutes later Dr. Brown is back. As I told your family, he says, your mom's heart is still going strong but her breathing. . .well, I think she's struggling.

When?

There's no way of telling, for sure. I'd be surprised if she makes it through the night, though.

Thank you, Dr. Brown.

~

A volunteer with a cart of ice water bottles passes Daniel as he nears the entrance to Rose Arbor. Visitors are crossing the parking lot as he leaves the building, a group of six that includes two adults and four younger people; one of the youngsters has a small dog on a leash in tow. Daniel decides to walk down the street toward the new apartments being constructed a half mile away. He wonders what it will be like in a few months, with traffic and noise and exhaust smells. He seems to remember reading in the newspaper about a zoning fight of some sort after the plan to build the apartments was announced, but the township apparently valued the potential property tax revenues more than it wanted to preserve the relative quiet of the neighborhood where Rose Arbor had been built only a few years ago.

Daniel marvels at the uncharacteristically pleasant October weather. Not a cloud in the brilliant blue sky. As he draws closer to the apartment complex he can hear the pop of pneumatic nail guns, and a generator, and the back-up signal of a delivery truck. At any other time he might stay to watch the men work, but he continues to walk, faster now, down the new road to where it crosses Drake, the Croyden School on the corner, a stretch of tidy homes beyond.

Daniel checks his watch, 4 p.m. His mother has been in Rose Arbor for only twenty-six hours.

At that moment his cell phone rings.

About the Authors

Jan Andersen

Jan Andersen is a Gemini, and her professional life reflects that duality. She owns two businesses.

On the one hand: She's been a communications professional, writer and editor for 25 years. She owns an organizational communication consulting firm, Beyond Words, which serves nonprofits, small and start-up companies, and government organizations. Jan has a gift for turning complex or technical material into "reader-friendly" language, which usually makes for happy readers.

On the other hand: Jan's main interest and life passion is health care, especially integrative and complementary medicine. Through her company, healingspace, she offers Usui Reiki, Healing Touch and other energy medicine-related health support services. She often uses essential oils in her practice and is a distributor for Young Living Essential Oils.

It all somehow works together and keeps her out of mischief—most of the time—well, usually. If you can't find her at work, go look in the woods somewhere.

Elizabeth Clark

She writes professionally and has done so since she was in college, specializing in light features and reviews for area newspapers.

She travels avocationally, has journeyed to 23 countries, can say "Cheers" and "Thank you" in about 50 languages and can turn a few naughty phrases in Norwegian.

She can roller-skate backwards, is a scrabble dynamo, still goes "trick or treating" and consumes 25 pounds of chocolate per year. She realizes how easy it is to make people smile or make someone's day and tries to do so as often as possible.

"Kudos to hospice for realizing this, too, and for providing such comfortable and loving end-of-life care. It was an honor to work on this project and encounter the fabulous people providing the loving care that makes Rose Arbor such a special place. I hope my loved ones get such tender treatment in their end days."

Patrick Crandell

I am currently attending law school, with the goal of eventually helping to craft public policy with the legislature. I am married (9 months now) to my beautiful wife, Jill. I wrote the essay as my own resolution to Chris' (or whatever I changed his name to) death. It wasn't easy coping with, and this was my expressive outlet.

I hope to make a significant contribution someday, make the world a better place. It's my goal, God has brought me to a place where I can work to make people's lives better. That's my driving force, to help whenever and wherever I'm needed. Law school is the first step; the second isn't clear yet.

Matt Crowe

I was born in May 1982, and I was twenty-one when I wrote this short story. I came across the opportunity to write for this project through my English professor, William Zinkus. I lost a grandfather and a great-grandmother to terminal cancer, and I can sympathize with the families of loved ones in Rose Arbor. After visiting the facility, I am a believer that its atmosphere has a presence unmatched by any health care facility that I have ever known. It emanates peace and calm, and it has a personality all its own.

I am a graduate of Western Michigan University, where I majored in English and Spanish. I married Danielle Hidalgo in August of 2005, and we reside in Kalamazoo, Michigan, where we met as undergrads at WMU. We will be leaving June 5 to serve as municipal development volunteers in the Peace Corps in El Salvador for the next two years and three months. My favorite author is Hemmingway, and my favorite book is *To Kill a Mockingbird*.

I love music, and I love the culture and art that thrives in the roots of the Kalamazoo community. I love the great outdoors—hunting, fishing, canoeing, hiking—and I love to write.

Diana Fox

Diana Fox is an award-winning screenwriter, playwright, author and freelance writer, having taught creative writing for 15 years. She has taught online, at Bainbridge Community College (Georgia), Kalamazoo Valley Community College, Kellogg Community College LifeLong Learning (Battle Creek), Western Michigan University, and Davenport University.

She received her MFA degree in Creative Writing from Western Michigan University in April 2006 and currently lives in Kalamazoo where she is working on a medieval novel.

Andrea Lanier

Born in the Year of the Dog, I'm a friendly stray inclined to collaborate rather than to obey a master. And like most strays, not having gone through life unscarred, I'm loyal to and grateful for the friends I make carefully and not always conventionally.

My amazing African-American husband of thirty years and my affinity for the spirit of Native Americans drew me west when I was a very young woman, but the essence of my philosophy for living has since drawn my spirit also toward the Far East at the same time drawing me into Nature wherever preserved in these incredible lands.

As a German immigrant with a passion for writing in English, I'm currently writing a book on my colored life with the hope that elements of my story might help others heal or mend. It was with that same hope that I wrote the story of Martin and Angela.

Dorothy LaRue

I believe everyone has interesting stories to tell and want to help people share those stories. We can learn so much from the experiences and perspectives of others.

I just moved from Kalamazoo to Metro Detroit *via* a five-month detour to the San Francisco Bay Area! Originally from New Hampshire, I lived in Boston for eight years, San Francisco for four and then Kalamazoo for six and a half. Going back to California provided valuable perspective on what my husband and I really want in life (and lifestyle) and where we want to be. Michigan is home and we are happy to be back. Life is full of unknowns for us now, but the challenges are where growth occurs and strength is gained.

The story I conveyed for this book underscores the importance of being grateful for all that we have, giving your all to each moment and trusting the Universe to take care of us.

Brenda Fettig Murphy

Brenda is a native of New York City who was transplanted to Kalamazoo over thirty years ago. She can still talk with a real New York accent, if the occasion or need presents itself.

Brenda draws and paints, plays tennis and golf, likes to ski, was once a member of an ice skating precision team, taught mathematics in high school and at the university level, has traveled to, and actually set foot on all seven continents and has a website, www.brendamurphyart.com, for her art work.

Her friends say she is compassionate and caring, artistic, adventurous, loyal, incredibly creative and has a wonderfully dry sense of humor.

She started volunteering for Hospice Care of Southwest Michigan at Rose Arbor in 1999, four years after her mother's death. She has been working on this book project since 2001.

Brenda feels boundless gratitude to all the people who contributed to this special book on so many different levels because without their efforts and support, it would not have been printed.

Elizabeth Cook Seering

Elizabeth grew up in the sleepy village of Pinckney, Michigan, before getting a Batchelor's degree in Practical Writing at Western Michigan University. She now lives with her husband, Matthew, in the beautiful coastal town of Wilmington, North Carolina.

Elizabeth adores going to church, reading anything she can get her hands on, being domesticated and playing with her two Bassett hounds, Roxy and Stuart. When she isn't working her day job—and even when she is—Elizabeth is busy thinking up new story ideas in the spirit of C.S. Lewis, Elisabeth Elliot and Francine Rivers.

When she started this story, it was as an assignment, but when she finished it, it was with a greater understanding of God's hands weaving all things together in death and beyond. *Dominus illuminatio mea.*

Beth Carroll VanHouten

I live in Traverse City with my husband, Adam.

I work for a children's book publisher.

I like to read and write.

I enjoy going to the beach; there are plenty to choose from here!

I enjoy hiking and camping.

William Zinkus

He was born in Toledo, Ohio, but has lived in Kalamazoo most of his life.

He's been a grocery store clerk, a U.S. Army medical corps-man, a liquor store manager, a self-employed house painter, a roofer, a dog trainer, a greenskeeper, a freelance writer and editor, a film critic, a college English teacher. . .to mention only a few of his many occupations.

He's owned twenty-eight different cars and trucks in his lifetime. He's the head golf coach at Hackett Catholic Central High School.

He loves to travel, fish, hike, bike, canoe, camp and ski cross-country, though not necessarily all at the same time.

He had difficulty thinking of interesting things about himself.

~

Living Well, Dying Well

Journal

To order more copies of

Living Well, Dying Well:
Stories from Rose Arbor Hospice

Each softcover copy is $15.95 with 25% discount for 10 or more copies.

copies _____ x _____ = $ _____

Shipping and Handling:
$3.00 for first book and
$1.50 for each additional book $ _____

Tax: Michigan residents,
add 6% sales tax $ _____

Checks payable to:
Hospice Care of Southwest Michigan

Mail order form and payment to:
Hospice Care of Southwest Michigan
222 North Kalamazoo Mall, Suite 100
Kalamazoo, Michigan 49007

Send book/s to (please print):

Name _____

Street _____

City _____ State/Prov _____

Zip _____ Phone _____

E-mail _____

For more information, call the Director of Community
Relations & Development at 269-345-0273.
www.hospiceswmi.org